"The Object Lessons series achieves something very close to magic: the books take ordinary—even banal—objects and animate them with a rich history of invention, political struggle, science, and popular mythology. Filled with fascinating details and conveyed in sharp, accessible prose, the books make the everyday world come to life. Be warned: once you've read a few of these, you'll start walking around your house, picking up random objects, and musing aloud: 'I wonder what the story is behind this thing?'"

Steven Johnson, author of *Where Good Ideas Come From* and *How We Got to Now*

"Object Lessons describes themselves as 'short, beautiful books,' and to that, I'll say, amen. . . . If you read enough Object Lessons books, you'll fill your head with plenty of trivia to amaze and annoy your friends and loved ones—caution recommended on pontificating on the objects surrounding you. More importantly, though . . . they inspire us to take a second look at parts of the everyday that we've taken for granted. These are not so much lessons about the objects themselves, but opportunities for self-reflection and storytelling. They remind us that we are surrounded by a wondrous world, as long as we care to look."

John Warner, *The Chicago Tribune*

"Besides being beautiful little hand-sized objects themselves, showcasing exceptional writing, the wonder of these books is that they exist at all . . . Uniformly excellent, engaging, thought-provoking, and informative."

Jennifer Bort Yacovissi, *Washington Independent Review of Books*

". . . edifying and entertaining . . . perfect for slipping in a pocket and pulling out when life is on hold."

Sarah Murdoch, *Toronto Star*

"For my money, Object Lessons is the most consistently interesting nonfiction book series in America."

Megan Volpert, *PopMatters*

"Though short, at roughly 25,000 words apiece, these books are anything but slight."

Marina Benjamin, *New Statesman*

"[W]itty, thought-provoking, and poetic . . . These little books are a page-flipper's dream."

John Timpane, *The Philadelphia Inquirer*

"The joy of the series, of reading *Remote Control*, *Golf Ball*, *Driver's License*, *Drone*, *Silence*, *Glass*, *Refrigerator*, *Hotel*, and *Waste* (more titles are listed as forthcoming) in quick succession, lies in encountering the various turns through which each of their authors has been put by his or her object. As for Benjamin, so for the authors of the series, the object predominates, sits squarely center stage, directs the action. The object decides the genre, the chronology, and the limits of the study. Accordingly, the author has to take her cue from the *thing* she chose or that chose her. The result is a wonderfully uneven series of books, each one a *thing* unto itself."

Julian Yates, *Los Angeles Review of Books*

"The Object Lessons series has a beautifully simple premise. Each book or essay centers on a specific object. This can be mundane or unexpected, humorous or politically timely. Whatever the subject, these descriptions reveal the rich worlds hidden under the surface of things."

Christine Ro, *Book Riot*

". . . a sensibility somewhere between Roland Barthes and Wes Anderson."

Simon Reynolds, author of *Retromania: Pop Culture's Addiction to Its Own Past*

"My favourite series of short pop culture books"

Zoomer magazine

"Bloomsbury's Object Lessons series never misses"

The Millions

BOOKS IN THE SERIES

Air Conditioning by Hsuan L. Hsu
Alarm by Alice Bennett
Ballot by Anjali Enjeti
Barcode by Jordan Frith
Bicycle by Jonathan Maskit
Bird by Erik Anderson
Blackface by Ayanna Thompson
Blanket by Kara Thompson
Blue Jeans by Carolyn Purnell
Bookshelf by Lydia Pyne
Bread by Scott Cutler Shershow
Bulletproof Vest by Kenneth R. Rosen
Burger by Carol J. Adams
Cell Tower by Steven E. Jones
Cigarette Lighter by Jack Pendarvis
Coffee by Dinah Lenney
Compact Disc by Robert Barry
Doctor by Andrew Bomback
Doll by Maria Teresa Hart
Driver's License by Meredith Castile
Drone by Adam Rothstein
Dust by Michael Marder
Earth by Jeffrey Jerome Cohen and Linda T. Elkins-Tanton
Egg by Nicole Walker
Email by Randy Malamud
Environment by Rolf Halden
Exit by Laura Waddell
Eye Chart by William Germano
Fat by Hanne Blank
Glass by John Garrison
Golf Ball by Harry Brown
Fake by Kati Stevens
Football by Mark Yakich
Gin by Shonna Milliken Humphrey
Glasses by Adam Geczy
Glitter by Nicole Seymour
Grave by Allison C. Meier
Hair by Scott Lowe
Hashtag by Elizabeth Losh
High Heel by Summer Brennan
Hood by Alison Kinney
Hotel by Joanna Walsh
Hyphen by Pardis Mahdavi
Island by Julian Hanna
Jet Lag by Christopher J. Lee
Lawn by Giovanni Aloi
Luggage by Susan Harlan
Magazine by Jeff Jarvis
Magnet by Eva Barbarossa
Mask by Sharrona Pearl
Metronome by Matthew Birkhold
Microphone by Ralph Jones
Mushroom by Sara Rich
Newspaper by Maggie Messitt
Ocean by Steve Mentz
Office by Sheila Liming
Oil by Michael Tondre
OK by Michelle McSweeney
Password by Martin Paul Eve
Pencil by Carol Beggy
Perfume by Megan Volpert
Personal Stereo by Rebecca Tuhus-Dubrow
Phone Booth by Ariana Kelly
Pill by Robert Bennett
Political Sign by Tobias Carroll
Potato by Rebecca Earle
Pregnancy Test by Karen Weingarten
Pub by Philip Howell
Questionnaire by Evan Kindley
Recipe by Lynn Z. Bloom
Refrigerator by Jonathan Rees
Remote Control by Caetlin Benson-Allott
Restaurant by Brian Duff
Rust by Jean-Michel Rabaté
Saxophone by Mollie Hawkins
Sewer by Jessica Leigh Hester
Scream by Michael J. Seidlinger
Shipping Container by Craig Martin
Shopping Mall by Matthew Newton
Signature by Hunter Dukes
Silence by John Biguenet
Skateboard by Jonathan Russell Clark
Sock by Kim Adrian
Souvenir by Rolf Potts
Snack by Eurie Dahn
Snake by Erica Wright
Spacecraft by Timothy Morton
Space Rover by Stewart Lawrence Sinclair
Sticker by Henry Hoke
Stock Photo by Simona Supekar
Stroller by Amanda Parrish Morgan
Swimming Pool by Hsuan L. Hsu
Taco by Ignacio M. Sánchez Prado
Traffic by Paul Josephson
Tree by Matthew Battles
Trench Coat by Jane Tynan
Tumor by Anna Leahy
TV by Susan Bordo
Veil by Rafia Zakaria
Videotape by Oana Godeanu-Kenworthy
Waste by Brian Thill
Whale Song by Margret Grebowicz
Wine by Meg Bernhard
X-ray by Nicole Lobdell

OBJECTLESSONS

A book series about the hidden lives of ordinary things.

Series Editors:

Ian Bogost and Christopher Schaberg

In association with

Program
in Public Scholarship

Washington
University in St. Louis

Glasses

ADAM GECZY

BLOOMSBURY ACADEMIC
NEW YORK • LONDON • OXFORD • NEW DELHI • SYDNEY

BLOOMSBURY ACADEMIC
Bloomsbury Publishing Inc, 1359 Broadway, New York, NY 10018, USA
Bloomsbury Publishing Plc, 50 Bedford Square, London, WC1B 3DP, UK
Bloomsbury Publishing Ireland, 29 Earlsfort Terrace, Dublin 2, D02 AY28, Ireland

BLOOMSBURY, BLOOMSBURY ACADEMIC and the Diana logo are trademarks of Bloomsbury Publishing Plc

First published in the United States of America 2026

Series design by Alice Marwick
Cover illustration © Cristiano Siqueira / crisvector.com

Library of Congress Cataloging-in-Publication Data
Names: Geczy, Adam author
Title: Glasses / Adam Geczy.
Description: New York : Bloomsbury Academic, 2026. | Series: Object lessons | Includes bibliographical references and index.
Identifiers: LCCN 2026001604 | ISBN 9798765135556 paperback | ISBN 9798765135549 epdf | ISBN 9798765135563 ebook
Subjects: LCSH: Eyeglasses–Social aspects
Classification: LCC GT2370 .G43 2026 | DDC 391.4/4–dc23/eng/20260204
LC record available at https://lccn.loc.gov/2026001604

ISBN: PB: 9798765135556
ePDF: 9798765135549
eBook: 9798765135563

Series: Object Lessons

Typeset by Deanta Global Publishing Services, Chennai, India
Printed and bound in the United States of America

For product safety related questions contact productsafety@bloomsbury.com.

To my dear, eternally bespectacled friend, David

CONTENTS

ILLUSTRATIONS

INTRODUCTION

ROSE-COLORED GLASSES

In the 1964 film *Tomb of Ligeia*, based loosely on Edgar Allan Poe's tale, Verden Fell is a forlorn widower beset with an eye condition that leaves him wearing dark glasses outdoors, a metaphor for his infirmity, melancholy, and withdrawal from the world. Fell's glasses are blinkered, covering front and side, concealing any possible affect that his eyes may disclose. His covered eyes yield a deeper significance as the plot unfolds when seeing and believing become increasingly discordant. Fell's photosensitivity is the breach between him and reality until he is finally blinded by the cat that is supposed to be the incarnation of his deceased wife, Ligeia, leading to his doom.

I remember this film like I saw it yesterday, and most notably the sinister glasses. I saw it as a child of twelve or so one night at a sleepover at a friend's place. We snuck downstairs once his parents had gone to bed to see what was on for the Saturday late night movies special. This was where I got my first taste of Hammer and Alta Vista film productions—the sinister man made inscrutable by glasses hiding his eyes was seared into my consciousness forever. When I saw the film I was wearing glasses, which meant that, when my friend announced that the coast was clear, I rose up together with the action of grabbing my glasses that had been carefully folded beside my bed. It was an action that was natural enough and to which I never at the time gave a second thought. Prosaic as it was, it will probably have some credible resonance to those readers who wear glasses. These actions are instinctively superadded to the ones you had before you wore them. They become part of your normal bodily regime; they become part of you.

Apart from the other various situations that befall a teenage youth wearing glasses—the nagging burden of that thing on my nose, the uncomfortable sweatiness on a hot day, the grime, the occasional but regular ridicule, the need to take them off when getting into a fight, the visits to the optometrist, the imperfect hand-eye coordination—the most striking and lasting memory of all is the most germane to this book. In my teens I only needed to use glasses while reading, which meant they were otherwise kept in a case. Returning home at the end of a school day, I would typically need to cross a busy main road. One afternoon, after rushing between the traffic, too lazy to wait for the pedestrian lights, I realized my glasses case had fallen from my schoolbag. Without any hesitation I lunged onto the road to retrieve it but was abruptly made to recoil from a passing car which shattered it with an agonizingly piercing "thwak." My shock was less over the broken glasses than at my instincts: I had treated my glasses—blindly—as an appendage, as an extension of my body such that I would unthinkingly need to retrieve them if ever detached from them.

Most people heavily reliant on glasses will relate to this. Glasses become a function of their wholeness, the suturing point between their body and the world. Witness how a chronic myopic will spring to life when they put on their glasses. Or when you hesitate before recognizing them with their glasses off because you know them only with glasses. Or the telltale discomfort and momentary disorientation you feel when they adopt contact lenses: their faces seem too bare, divested, "nude."

The distinguished air of an adult wearing glasses rarely correlates to a youth. Glasses on the young are considered an unfortunate necessity to compensate for a defect that should typically only arise in later years. In adolescent years, some girls may have escaped the stigma, but scarcely the boys for whom glasses, full-time at least, were a sign of a lack of prowess and virility and a source of intermittent mockery. These corollaries, invidious as they are, have a germ of truth, because poor eyesight is a significant impediment, especially in ball and group sports. And by extension, these deficiencies imply retreat into indoor, booking pursuits that are deemed comparatively effete and, for a boy, effeminizing. It is a harbinger of a draft-dodger and a coward. For a girl, glasses are a sure sign that she won't get the guy and is consigned to compromise with her choice of mate, or worse, spinsterhood. Or at least that is how it used to be.

Maybe all these stereotypes have faded a little now. As the 1980s song by Huey Lewis has it, "It's hip to be square." Glasses are full of connotations and semantics, but they are also seamless with everyday life. That many of the negative connotations have diminished in our time is attributable, in my view, to three main factors. The first is that for most of those reading this book, we are in a post-industrial society where the premiums are less on labor and more on technology and services. Reorienting work has had the imperceptible, but still decisive effect of making us rethink the worker. Fewer of us work in the fields than those that sit at desks before computers, which means that you are more prone to wearing glasses, even if they are meant to mitigate the glare of the screen. At the end of the last century, people still distinguished between manual labor and blue- and white-collar work. Notice that we don't hear these terms very often anymore. Wearing glasses no longer implies that you've shied away from work that is physical.

The second is that we live in a universe of prostheses: physical and mental add-ons. We feel naked without them. It will increasingly be the case that someone wearing glasses in public may not necessarily be shortsighted but is using them as an extra-intelligence tool.

Finally, the third reason is that people are living longer. By dint of more people past middle age proportionate to the young in the history of the species, there will be more people who need to wear glasses due to natural macular degeneration. Once free of adolescence, wearing glasses assumes a miraculous change of fortune. The link to nerdiness is transformed into signs of thoughtfulness and integrity. To wear glasses without demur means that you accept your age with good grace. They are also useful appendages to hide behind, affording you minor distance, and giving you pause when you take them off. Not being able to see so well is not entirely a disadvantage, for it may offer temporary reprieve.

On closer inspection, the expression, "Looking at the world with rose-colored glasses" is less self-evident than you may first think. The common meaning is to see the world in an unrealistically positive light. But to wear glasses is to see the world better than without them. Verden Fell wore his as a buffer to protect his shattered nerves from a cruel world. Even the nerd who has little choice to wear glasses does so because life is harder without them. Pop stars wear dark shades to look cool, as a barrier between them and their fans, and to generate an air of mystique. When we don't see them on scholars and bookish types, we may feel disappointed, maybe even defrauded. The real alchemy is reached when a celebrity dons a pair: in covering up such beautiful features we are made to long for them even more. Or that they are so confident that they have transcended vanity, an attractiveness that comes from insouciance. It also marks a certain coming of age that implies a new layer of dignity over the glamor.

The contradiction in glasses is that they can be both at the service of seeing more and of seeing less, but always with the goal of seeing better. To the consternation of the expression "keep your eyes peeled," glasses can make the world sharper, enhancing the field of vision, or they can make it dimmer to desensitize against too many stimuli. Then there are the glasses of the blind which save all those who do see from the discomfort of a vacant stare while also reminding them that the gaze is inward, and a new array of senses has been brought into play. In this respect, the dark glasses of the blind are closer to the digitally assisted eyewear of the future, for these are an assisted blindness to the immediate, tangible world for the sake of seeing beyond and behind it.

1 LOOKING BETTER

The relationship between children and glasses is rarely a harmonious one. From the outset, glasses signal deficiency. A child wearing them often evokes sympathy, as if their vision impairment somehow limits their capacity for play, adventure, or agency. They are seen as fragile, timid—hemmed in by a quiet debility. Yet these assumptions can be startlingly upended. There's a jolt of surprise when a bespectacled child defies expectations—running wild, loud, unruly. And there's a different kind of disappointment when a child with glasses turns out not to be especially bright, as if the visual aid had promised intellectual compensation that never arrived.

Much of this reflection is drawn from personal experience, though I'll keep the autobiographical tone to a minimum. Glasses, for me, offered not just clearer sight but a skewed perspective—both literally and socially. They taught me early on how much appearances matter, and how even the most compassionate people are quick to judge. In hindsight, I'm grateful. Being slightly on the outside gave me a different vantage point.

For children who wear glasses full-time, the reality is often frustrating. Glasses slip, fall, break—and when they break, you're the one in trouble. They impose a kind of caution that runs counter to the spirit of childhood. When they fall off, the world becomes a fog, and you're often relegated to the sidelines, watching others play while you squint from a distance.

Before adolescence, glasses are chosen for you. Your only role is to comply, usually to please your parents. But as you grow older, a new layer of resentment emerges. You begin to compare yourself to peers who aren't burdened by this visible marker of limitation. Even as more children join your ranks—part-time wearers or those with newly discovered vision issues—the sense of difference lingers. Fashion enters the equation. Glasses become not just a necessity but a statement. My advice? Don't chase the most expensive frames. Find the coolest look at the lowest cost.

There's no universal moment when glasses stop being a source of embarrassment and start becoming a badge of character. But it happens. As the rough-and-tumble of childhood gives way to more reflective teenage years, glasses begin to carry different connotations. They may suggest thoughtfulness, introspection, even allure. The stereotype of the "geek" gives way to the possibility of the "intellectual," the "mysterious," or the "artsy." For some, glasses become part of their identity—so much so that they feel unrecognizable without them.

In this way, glasses can mark a quiet evolution: from burden to expression, from stigma to style. They may still carry the weight of old associations, but they also offer a way to stand out, to signal depth, and to shape how others see you—just as they help you see the world more clearly.

Glasses have long carried symbolic weight, often standing in for deeper ideas about perception, knowledge, and human limitation. They suggest not only a physical impairment but also a metaphorical one—the inability to see things as they truly are. Yet, paradoxically, they also imply the opposite: enhanced insight, deeper understanding, and intellectual acuity.

Shakespeare makes several references to glasses in this vein. In *King Lear*, Gloucester, tricked by his son Edmund, remarks, "Come, if it be nothing, I shall not need spectacles" (1.2.34), equating the need for glasses with the need to discern truth. In *As You Like It*, Jacques's famous "Seven Ages of Man" speech marks spectacles as a sign of decline: "The sixth age shifts / Into the lean and slipper'd pantaloon / With spectacles on nose and pouch on side" (2.7.1037). Spectacles here are not tools of wisdom but emblems of frailty and old age.

Elsewhere, Shakespeare uses glasses to underscore irony or blindness. In *Henry VI*, the king mocks Salisbury's age and weakness: "What, wilt thou on thy death-bed play the ruffian, / And seek for sorrow with thy spectacles?" (5.1.3151). In *Much Ado About Nothing*, Benedick boasts, "I can see yet without spectacles and I see no such matter" (1.1.170), dismissing both literal and metaphorical insight. And in *The Winter's Tale*, Leontes scolds Camillo for failing to see the obvious, saying, "Your eye-glass is thicker than a cuckold's horn" (1.2.369)—a biting metaphor for willful blindness.

Spectacles as object and metaphor take us to the slippery meaning of "seeing." Seeing is more than sight; it is perceiving, identifying, understanding, demystifying, judging. To need an extra device to help you understand is to underscore your imperfection, but the opposite side is just as true. Hence a persistent cultural tension: glasses are both aids and admissions of failure. To wear them is to acknowledge imperfection, yet also to claim a kind of superiority—an ability to see more clearly, more deeply. They mark the wearer as someone who looks harder, thinks longer, and perhaps understands more.

This symbolism has endured. Glasses remain shorthand for the scholar, the bookworm, the introspective thinker, the savant. They suggest a life of the mind, a gaze turned inward or focused intently on the world. In this way, they are not just tools but talismans—objects that carry the weight of centuries of cultural meaning.

The origins of glasses are as layered and contested as the lenses themselves. Their invention is typically traced to the mid-thirteenth century, often credited to the English polymath Roger Bacon. Yet competing claims emerge from Italy, where both Alessandro della Spina, a Pisan monk, and Salvino degli Armati, a Florentine nobleman, are said to have pioneered early spectacles. This ambiguity—Florence versus

Pisa—reflects not only historical rivalry but also the elusive nature of innovation itself.

Umberto Eco playfully revisits this debate in *The Name of the Rose*, where the protagonist Guglielmo, a monk and sleuth, shows off his treasured glasses, attributing them to Salvino. The monastery's glazier counters, citing Brother Jordan and his 1313 funeral oration crediting Spina. Such literary nods underscore how glasses, even in fiction, are bound up with questions of origin, authority, and perception.

Before these framed lenses, vision enhancement came in the form of "beryl moons"—glass globules or reading stones placed directly on texts to magnify them. Ptolemy's *Optics* mentions such devices, and there are claims—though now discredited—that Marco Polo encountered eyeglasses in China. The earliest confirmed spectacles, as we know them, likely emerged in central Italy around 1290, aided by the advanced glassmaking techniques of Murano artisans in Venice. By 1320, glasses were common enough in Venice to warrant their own guild.

These early spectacles were rudimentary: two lollipop-shaped lenses joined by a rivet, held up to the eyes or perched on the nose like a pince-nez (literally "squeeze nose"). As many of the earliest pictures show, these were typically made of two lollipop-shaped pieces joined by a rivet. Frames were crafted from metal, wood, horn, shell, or bone. Because of the skill required to grind lenses, glasses were prized possessions—symbols of privilege as much as tools of clarity. Bifocals are credited to Benjamin Franklin who was both nearsighted (myopia) and farsighted (hyperopia). For his time, such an invention would have been thought of as both brilliant and highly eccentric, like wearing an unfamiliar crafted apparatus over the eyes.

The tyrannical friar Girolamo Savonarola (1452–98) affirmed that glasses could be affixed to the head by a ribbon, while eyeglasses as we know them today, supported by the nose and ears, are accredited to Edward Scarlett, a London optician and instrument maker who introduced them in the 1720s. (Astigmatism, the condition of rotational asymmetry of the cornea, was only identified in 1801 by the polymath Thomas Young, better known for deciphering Egyptian hieroglyphics using the Rosetta Stone.) Until only recently in the twentieth century, glasses were generic, not made-to-order according to the prescription of an ophthalmologist. Rather, they were more like the kind sold in graded strengths that we today find in pharmacies or drugstores.

If "glasses" in English has an innocuous etymology (we are not alone, for instance the Italian is *occhiali*), the word in Germanic languages—in German *Brille* (they also have *Gläser*), Danish *briller*, Dutch *bril*—is considerably more telling as to the early days of corrective lenses. The Medieval Germanic *Berille*, adapted from the Latin *beryllus*, was the general word for shiny (whence the French *briller* to shine) crystals, some of which we made into reading aids. Skilled Flemish stone cutters who fashioned stones specifically for reading were known as *de bril* after the stones they shaped. Glasses as we know them were of glass, not semi-precious stone, and became widespread because they were cheaper and more amenable than carrying a stone in your pocket.

Pliny the Elder, in his chapter on precious stones in *Natural History,* cites the *smaragdus,* now better known as emeralds, used for reflection when flat or assisting with shortsightedness when concave. "The Emperor Nero used to view the combats of the gladiators upon a *smaragdus.*"[1] Apart from these isolated cases, a burning question may prey upon the mind of the curious antiquarian, namely that given their demonstrated technological ingenuity, why the Romans did not turn their attentions to assisting those with diminished vision. They were, after all, a culture that venerated old age: despite not always adhering to this rule, entry to the senate could only be over 40 (*senatus* means "old man"), at the very time when macular degeneration begins to set in and vision declines, and where the generic senescent squint sets in. (Presbyopia, the term for ocular degeneration due to age, derives from the Greek *presbus* for "old man.")

Digging down into this counterfactual, we can speculate that the literate were the wealthier members of society who would also have had slaves who came from all levels of society. Elite Romans had literate slaves who ran the household and conducted duties such as monitoring everyday expenses. This meant that if you could not read for yourself, you could afford the luxury of having someone else read for you. Educated slaves in at least the time of the ancient Greeks were relied upon to teach the children of upper-class families. (The Stoic philosopher Epictetus began life as a slave and was sought out by Hadrian.) Such privileges were no longer available in the Middle Ages where resources were uneven and, when slaves were held, they were unlikely to be literate and scarcely used for anything other than manual labor.[2] (A more recent evolution from excess to utility is maybe the wristwatch, the sibling prosthesis of glasses. Men were expected to have a fob watch which would be kept in the vest or waistcoat, and when watches began to be worn on one's person in the nineteenth century it was by women. The effeminacy associated with wristwatches was dispelled in the First World War when keeping time with a fob proved far too impractical.) We have no evidence at all for this of course but we do know that there are always social and material conditions for the appearance of a thing, and it is a pleasant idea to suppose that the appearance of the medium for aiding perception was delayed by a different form of perception, that of status.

Today this has somewhat reversed, but still only relatively recently. Think about cinema from the silent years to the golden age. The only characters wearing glasses were secondary: the professors, the grandpa, the nerd scientist. Or by the sinister villain, where glasses marked him out in his abnormality, the telltale hint of a deeper dissonance in his soul. And they were almost always men. When worn by a woman not noticeably of older age, she was a spinster. Glasses were the death knell of sex appeal. These were the peripheral figures of the world, not the star performers. Those who needed help to see were socially less visible. This is all consistent with the times, since still in the 1930s glasses were classed as "medical appliances."[3]

Proportionately fewer women wore glasses. Occasional paintings in the eighteenth century depict some, but these tend to be older women in subsidiary roles in the overall composition, either accompanying a musical ensemble, reading a book, or hunched over knitting or embroidery. By the nineteenth century, images of women wearing glasses began to surface a bit more, but they remained unusual. That rarity makes them quite striking, as the viewer notices the spectacles amid the reigning convention of comeliness. In these cases, glasses appeared as lorgnettes or sometimes as monocles, accessories attached to a golden thread or chain and not placed on the face. Only with photography, which was more geared toward an accurate likeness, do glasses begin to appear on women sitters, but these figures sometimes adopt a melancholy quality, as if they have resigned themselves to a lonely life. Are the glasses the reason why?

Hollywood reinforced these tropes. We only need to look again at the official photographic portraits of the stars of the golden age: none have glasses. Gregory Peck donned glasses in his famous role as the attorney Atticus Finch in the 1962 film adaptation of *To Kill a Mockingbird*, their effectiveness being an added accessory to how the actor was normally seen, making him out to be not only a man of balanced judgment but also one absent of vanity. Until then, glasses were for the quirky and comic—as with Harold Lloyd's horn-rimmed glasses in the silent era of the 1910s and 1920s (more on him later)—or the old. But even when the central roles were older men, good eyesight seemed part of their longevity, as in the grand old man of early cinema in *Goodbye, Mr. Chips* (1939, played by Robert Donat), although the 1969 version played by Peter O'Toole has him in horn-rimmed round glasses, to add to his vulnerable amiability.

Peck's character was high in the mind of popular memory, and it is a case that tends to embody the celebrity paradox of glasses. It was precisely the celebrities known for their physical beauty and sex appeal that could afford to be seen and photographed wearing glasses: James Dean, Brigitte Bardot, Ingrid Bergman, Marilyn Monroe. Marilyn's marriage to the bespectacled Arthur Miller was such a talking point of why the most desired woman in the world would accept a man with what was still viewed by many as having an emasculating characteristic.

Now, "medical appliances" have become "eyewear," and in the relatively new area of Disability Studies, glasses are the cornerstone where design and disability meet.[4] This may sound like nonsense and it may take a moment to think about how glasses normalize disability, as their universality cancels out any sense of that being so. They are also big business. It is hard not to see that the stigma on glasses became more relaxed with the growing sophistication of plastic technology and polymer chemistry. Fast and cheap to make, glasses were a profitable commodity. Just as we were told that breakfast was the most important meal of the day to make us eat cornflakes, by the 1970s glasses began to be cool. Think Elvis in the later, chubby years. Now no self-respecting fashion house is without a line of eyewear, from frames to shades.

The rare historical exceptions in paintings have less to do with fashion statements and more with the assertiveness of sight as bound to insight and discernment. Another casual scan of portraits before the twentieth century will reveal remarkably few people wearing glasses, and heaven forbid that women be represented with them! There are a few from the seventeenth century from Spain of notables in Spain and Portugal where in some the pince-nez is especially pronounced, and the number begins to step up in the nineteenth. The most familiar to us is maybe that of Franz Schubert, as there is a stunning likeness of him at the age of seventeen wearing a pair that are like conductors of his own intensity. The paucity of images of people wearing glasses in the eighteenth century is maybe a topic for another day, but suffice it to say that overall appearance and elegance were premium aspirations. It was only after the Romantics that the idea of an enigmatic inner life became a matter for consideration, and glasses were literally the lenses into inner depths, while equally being the barrier, or threshold between what people can really know about one another. (This theme of glasses as being both a gateway to greater subjective access as well as a barrier will be discussed later.) Glasses could also be a useful asset to the dandy that sprang up in the early nineteenth century, as they could be used, especially when attached with a ribbon, as a useful affectation in florid gestures of removing and replacing. The monocle was especially suited to this kind of behavior and for affecting quizzical and disapproving looks.

This infrequency in the eighteenth century makes the rare cases especially notable, such as Franklin and my favorite, bar none, Jean-Baptiste-Siméon Chardin (Figure 1.1). His self-portraits (at least four of them) now make far more sense to me writing this book. Every one of them shows him wearing a *lorgnon* (the more commonly used word in France for "pince-nez").

Figure 1.1 is him in 1775, aged 76. He stares out at us without perturbation, with a self-possessed fixity unencumbered by arrogance or false modesty. The even-handedness and purity of the stare are captivating. His eyes are intent and unflinching, asking nothing of us. He is wearing a head wrap to warm his head (far more hygienic than a louse-ridden wig) and which also helps keep in place a visor, relatable to our baseball caps but which was used to temper the light emitted from a raised window or skylight while painting. I am unaware of any similar depictions in works of this or any other time, so together with the glasses the exceptions keep multiplying. The limited color range suggests an uninterest in any flamboyance or artifice. He is an old man, but his faculties announce themselves to us undimmed.

What makes all these points so relevant is that Chardin devoted his life to looking at things surely, keenly, frankly. It is hard to dislike his work, and to call him among your favorite artists hardly makes you a member of a small group.

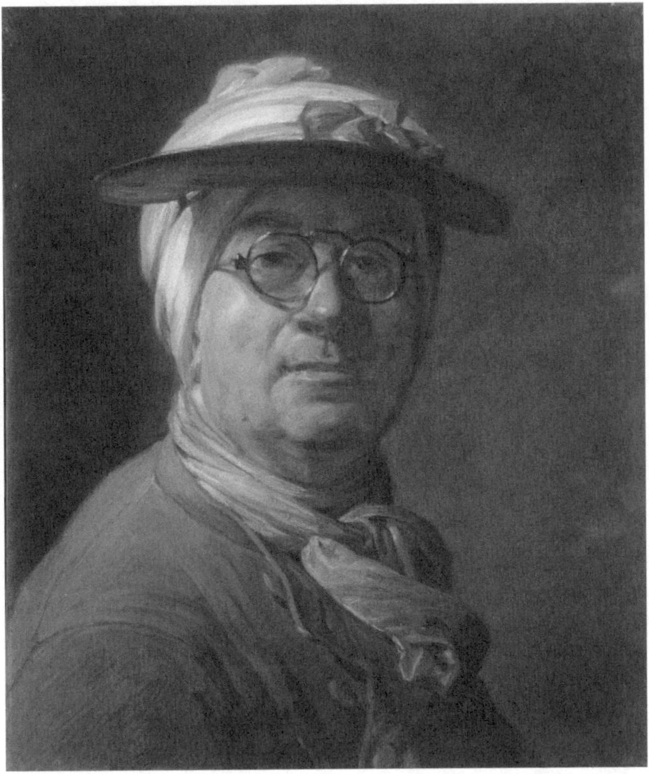

FIGURE 1.1 Jean-Baptiste Siméon Chardin, Self-Portrait with an Eyeshade, 1775, pastel, public domain

Chardin's gifts as a painter were quickly recognized in his own lifetime as a master of depicting arranged domestic objects and food with a mastery of light and handling of paint. Although he did produce modest figure paintings, it is for still lifes for which his name has become synonymous. The lighting is soft, in some even muted, and the paint is applied in numerous layers adding to the tangible textures of humble fruits and *faences*, brioches and berries. Chardin is only known for 200 paintings, which means an average of four a year. Legend has it that he would close himself up in his studio for hours at a time applying himself selflessly to his work to give his subjects and arrangements a second life. In short, this was a person who looked, intensely and attentively. This was an artist who gave his subjects and his painting the strictest attention, and attention that bordered on veneration. His self-portrait declares this by announcing not only "Here I am" but also "I am placed on this earth to look." Where it was customary for painters to capture themselves at work with the tools of their trade—palette, paints, easel—Chardin dispenses with all of that and gives us only his gaze while also announcing without hesitation that this most valued quality, sight, is made possible with glasses. The naturalness and integrity of his paintings and the frankness of his stare are products of a humble prosthesis, for which he seems to be grateful.

In the annals of human discovery and visual prostheses, I could delve into Galileo and Newton, but, tempting as it is, I don't want to take this discussion too far *off piste*. The story to rival Chardin's is possibly that of Baruch Spinoza, the great Dutch philosopher who lived a century before. A few likenesses of him survive, none of them with glasses, but the most important detail is that before he became renowned as a philosopher and before he died in 1677, Spinoza eked out a modest living as a lens grinder, assisted by the largesse of a few friends. Since the early days of lens manufacturing in fourteenth-century Venice, lens grinding became a skill unto itself, and one that was zealously taken up by the technology-minded labor market of the Low Countries by the seventeenth century.

As a result of the radicality of his ideas, Spinoza's earlier life was riven by hostility, including his expulsion or *herem* from the Jewish community when only twenty-three in an explosively worded writ. Spinoza's sin was to have viewed the universe as not simply emanating from a single entity but rather arguing that God inheres in the world in an unthinkably intricate set of interconnected causes and effects. Spinoza, the maker and polisher of lenses for glasses and telescopes, afforded a way of thinking that was beyond appearances toward how they worked upon one another. Writing in the early nineteenth century, the poet Heinrich Heine proclaimed that "[a]ll our present-day philosophers, possibly without knowing it, look through glasses that Baruch Spinoza ground."[5] In this light, glasses become emblems of intellectual humility and aspiration. They remind us that clarity often requires correction, that understanding is aided by tools—whether optical or conceptual. They are prosthetics of perception, extending our reach into the world and into ourselves.

Spinoza's example helps us to think of glasses as both material and metaphorical. On the one hand, they are the (now) everyday facilitators to unobstructed vision. On the other hand, philosophy and wisdom are lenses that enable us to navigate a cruel and inconsistent world with greater ease and acuity, and at best grant us closer, swifter access to clarity of vision, which in this case can also mean the beauty of better understanding.

2 LOOKING SMART

Ironically, the first known painting anywhere in the world of someone wearing glasses is inaccurate, which speaks powerfully to the association of glasses with mental aptitude. This is Tomaso of Modena's depiction of Hugh of Saint-Cher in 1352, who is shown hunched over a book, deep in study. He wears a pair of *bésicles*, the early form of pince-nez (the French language seems to have a monopoly stake in this item), which had become commonplace for Tomaso but had not yet materialized in Hugh's lifetime (*c.* 1200–1263). Tomaso can be forgiven for this, given the marginal gap of some thirty years, but his portrait is a powerful statement of the need to incorporate glasses in images to emphasize cleverness. Glasses, even then, had begun to signify intellect, study, and insight. Hugh, also known as Cardinal Hugues de Provence, was an erudite and studious theologian remembered for his distinction between the limitless potency of God and the conditional potency of kings. Intended to persuade more than document, Tomaso's painting makes us see that it did not take long for glasses' association with intelligence to take hold after their inception. But what this error also helps to articulate is that the association is far from accurate and can be used as a facile mask for what is lacking.

Glasses, not sunglasses, have a general tendency to make the wearer look intelligent, in affirmation or exaggeration. This tendency is closely linked to the perception that the wearer is more inept at physical activities than those who do not wear glasses. Glasses presupposing cleverness is an even more lasting cliché than glasses and old age because the old may be less mentally agile, but they are deemed wiser, so the link tenaciously persists regardless. But do glasses presuppose smarts or do smarts presuppose glasses? This is not a gratuitous question because it leads to the ramifying belief that wearers of glasses are less physically able. To start with the first premise: being more intelligent than most, the capacity to grasp complex ideas, process information quickly and in wide format, and the thirst for knowledge naturally leads to devouring large amounts of information. Traditionally this meant being hunched over books, now squinting before mobile devices, iPads, or computer screens. Irrespective of the case, these activities in excess tax the eyes (and may also lead to rounded shoulders). All of this is fairly straightforward. It's a causal narrative.

But then there is the child or youth who wants to run with his or her friends and gets infrequent headaches or dizziness, falters in walking a straight line, has difficulty in singling out objects, or cannot catch a ball, defectively doing what any innocent child thinks is second nature. Hopefully, they will get their eyes checked, and if that's the problem, glasses prescribed. Then they face the first social contradiction of their life. With their vision restored and with it the problems corrected, they are quickly alerted to the fragile fact that they now wear their debility (or disability, as the new language allows) written across their face. You are not like other children; you are now "four eyes." (I realize that my sensitivity as a grammarian, or semantic OCD, came at an early age because since very young, I couldn't quite get this slur as I insisted that the extra lenses were not eyes.)

It takes an unusually stubborn and rambunctious child to get beyond this. But even the child who wants to hang upside down from the monkey bars or lead the charge in the lunchtime football game will face immediate difficulty: the glasses will fly off, even break, and he or she is reduced to the same state as before, a minus one. They soon get adept at slotting back fallen lenses. If the glasses break, then there are the usual reprisals at home. Children of unwealthy single parents will be flagellated with guilt. Eventually, many kids just see bowing out of risky encounters with their friends as the easiest option, and casual retreat becomes a habit. It is easier to retire to the private space of books—or today it may be being glued to a device staring at YouTube. Either way, glasses force an osmosis of weakened activity that shunts one into more modest pursuits. It may accelerate smarter people into bookish behavior. Having intellectual gifts to whatever degree and being made prematurely to develop them is a consolation, for having glasses and being dim is worse still and rather pathetic. Being dumb and looking smart only emphasizes the lack. Stupidity is not always a want of intelligence, though, but maybe that is the bigger disability.

My own relationship with glasses began at the age of four, thanks to a toy. It was a Fisher Price View-Master—a plastic relic of the 1970s that now qualifies as "vintage" on eBay. This was a plastic eyepiece that held a circular disk, usually of paper and colored cells around its periphery that would slot into a cavity above. Directed to a light source, with the device over the eyes, you could navigate a narrative, typically a truncated version from a children's book—*Sesame Street*, *Caspar the Friendly Ghost* or a more traditional fairy tale like *Snow White* (the visuals adapted from the first great animated feature of 1937) by clicking a latch to the side. It was captivating analogue VR, or primitive proto-VR, and its charm was in its clunkiness because you had to fill in the rest with your own imaginative work.

But that enchantment came with a cost. After hours of peering into those tiny windows of fantasy, it became clear that something was wrong with my vision. I had pronounced monocular dominance—one eye doing all the work while the other drifted inward. The View-Master, ironically, helped reveal that I wasn't seeing the world as I should.

What followed was a series of interventions: two eye surgeries, adhesive patches over my dominant eye, and, of course, glasses. At five years old, I became the child with thick lenses and a lens patch—an image that elicited quiet sympathy from adults and casual cruelty from peers. I hated it.

All of this helped to register in me a particular combination of sympathy and contempt for non-adult wearers of glasses. These are to do with the anxieties over the runts of the litter who would not have been able to withstand pre-technological societies, immortalized by the character Piggy in William Golding's *Lord of the Flies*. The character of Piggy, fat, bespectacled, and asthmatic, is the embodiment of physical vulnerability and intellectual clarity. He is the voice of reason, the keeper of knowledge, and the only one who understands the importance of order. But he is also the first to be mocked, marginalized, and ultimately destroyed.

Piggy's glasses are more than a medical device—they are the group's only means of starting a fire, the literal spark of civilization. But they are also a target. The other boys don't just steal the glasses; they symbolically reject what they represent: rationality, restraint, and the uncomfortable truths of adulthood. When the glasses are shattered, so too is the last hope for order. Piggy's death follows soon after, a brutal silencing of intellect in favor of brute force.

Watching the film adaptation as a child, I couldn't help but wonder: would I be Piggy? Would my glasses mark me as expendable in a world stripped of rules? The question lingered, unsettling and formative. Piggy's fate is a cautionary tale—not just about the collapse of civilization, but about the fragility of those who see too clearly in a world that prefers not to look.

Writing in 1954, Golding would also certainly have had in mind the persecution of the Jews, a people traditionally prohibited from keeping land who as a result flourished as educated burghers, the bespectacled civic class, not the propertied warrior elite. The cultivation of the urban Jewry was envied and stigmatized as cowardice, although the limitations imposed on them were conveniently ignored. The Jewish people have always been known for being an especially clever people. For example, some of the most famous Jewish artists and intellectuals of *fin-de-siècle* Vienna wore glasses. Freud and Mahler come to mind immediately, as well as Alfred Adler and Stefan Zweig. It is notable that prominent women of the same era are not depicted wearing glasses.

For the stereotype, Mahler was a particularly fine case. Small in stature and of smoldering intensity, in his late 30s in 1897 he was made director of the main opera theater in Vienna, the Hofoper (now Staatsoper), a colossal organizational task which left him little time for his own music composition. Despite the burden of his professional duties, Mahler's constitution was fragile, being prone to migraines and hemorrhoids. This may be a coincidence, but it all chimes well with the glasses-wearer as having subpar physiology. The duality of brilliance and bodily limitation resonates with the broader cultural narrative around glasses, seen both as tools of enhancement and signs of deficiency. Mahler's case suggests that the two are not mutually exclusive. His glasses were not just corrective; they were emblematic of a deeper truth that genius often comes wrapped in vulnerability, and that the mind's reach may exceed the body's grasp.

A contemporary caricature of his frenetic, flamboyant conducting style leaves little room for doubting that he was a man of enormous sensitivity and intellect (Figure 2.1). In the picture, his glasses are very much part of his body and demeanor, and we see only the blank lenses, not his eyes, which in the language of modern comics, is a component of his "superpower." Without them, he couldn't function.

This example helps to show that glasses can unleash some hidden potential, a conduit to a potency formerly in abeyance. If Mahler represents the tortured genius behind the conductor's baton, John le Carré's George Smiley is his literary counterpart in the shadows of espionage. John le Carré's intelligence officer is the antithesis of the action hero: short, plump, physically unremarkable, and perpetually obscured behind thick glasses. Introduced as someone "not naturally equipped for hurrying in the rain" because "[h]is legs were short, his gait anything but agile, his dress costly," he is anything but frail and not someone disposed to smiling.[1] Wiley (rhymes with "Smiley"), methodical, and of mercurial cunning, Smiley is a senior intelligence officer for Britain at the height of the Cold War in the 1970s, emerging from forced retirement after a botched mission in Czechoslovakia that led to the torture of an agent. In *Tinker, Tailor, Soldier, Spy*, the first of the "Karla Trilogy," he is tasked with finding the Soviet mole that might have led to the earlier capture. The rain in the scene where he first enters "had formed in fat, unbanishable drops on the thick lenses of his spectacles, forcing him alternately to lower or throw back his head."[2]

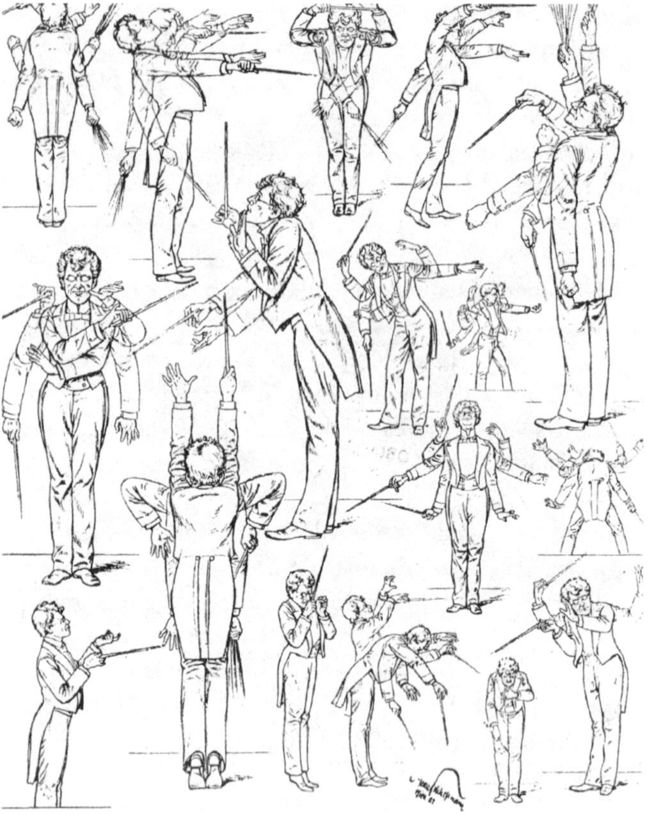

FIGURE 2.1 Caricature of Mahler conducting from the magazine, *Fliegende Blätter*, 1901, public domain

Smiley's glasses are central to his identity as a watcher, a thinker, a strategist. They are also a partition between his private feelings and his outward neutrality. Smiley's glasses are the tools of a man who sees what others miss, who survives not by strength but by intellect. And in this, Smiley joins a long tradition of bespectacled figures whose power lies not in their physicality, but in their ability to observe, analyze, and prevail.

This is made all the more pronounced on the occasions when he cleans his glasses on his tie, the mannerism for which he will become best known. In these brief intervals his cool detachment gives way to the vulnerability of the body:

> From the outset of this meeting, Smiley had assumed for the main a Buddha-like inscrutability from which neither Tarr's story nor the rare interjections of Lacon and Guillam could rouse him. He sat leaning back with his short legs bent, head forward, and plump hands linked across his generous stomach. His hooded eyes had closed behind his thick glasses. His only fidget was to polish his glasses on the silk lining of his tie, and when he did this his eyes had a soaked, naked look that was embarrassing to those who caught him at it.[3]

For those who are identified as indivisible from glasses, that short interval when they are publicly removed is where human nakedness and fragility are revealed to the discomfort of all who witness it. Those of us who relate to this on either side of the lens will recall the short moment of excruciating unease at what seems a voluntary humiliation. Why this is so is possibly because the transition occurs so instantly and so casually that its suddenness serves as a routine reminder of how quickly we can become unmasked and that our defenses are only ever temporary. There is always some moment of the day when we are naked, analogous to the unwelcome reminder that we will all one day die, departing as we began, as body, and body only.

In the television and film adaptations of the book, the character of Smiley fares a great deal better than his written description as fat and ungainly. In the 1979 BBC television series, he is played by Alec Guinness, and in the 2011 film by Gary Oldman, which assumes a fair amount of poetic license for the vehicle of the screen over the page. Some ten minutes into the film, just after Smiley has been placed into retirement, he makes his way to an optometrist. After a close-up of him in the ophthalmic brace for eye-testing, he re-emerges with new eyeglasses, the horn-rimmed of old replaced by a heavier, square style highly redolent of the 1970s. The implication is clear: his departure from the Circus (as the branch is called) has afforded him an alternative perspective which will prove to be effective when he returns and successfully unearths the mole.

As if in assurance of this connection with glasses and adept spying is seen around thirty minutes later with Prideaux, the agent formerly almost killed, now teaching at an all-boys school. He has taken a new boy in the class under his wing—squat, chubby, with bug-eyed glasses. After Prideaux gets his name (Bill), he asks the boy, "What are you good at?" getting the reply, "Nothing, sir." "You're a good watcher, though, eh?" adds Prideaux, "Us loners always are. 'Best watcher in the unit, Bill Roach is our bet.' As long as he has his specs on, right?" "Yes, sir."[4] Prideaux doesn't wear glasses, but he knows the type who does: the boy consigned to the margins who, by dint of being made to feel useless, becomes the silent judge of others. Children with glasses are seldom in the thick of it, but because of this they might have some insights about others who are and take it for granted. By extension, it may just make such a pariah end up doing the dirty work of gathering intelligence to keep the luckier people safe. (In the later adaptation of Le Carré's *Our Kind of Traitor* [2016], the only character wearing glasses is the Smiley spin-off, MI6 agent Hector [Damian Lewis], which are deep red and have sharply raised tips to convey a feline craftiness.)

What is striking across the uneven fabric of popular culture is just how few instances there are where someone wearing glasses is at the epicenter of the action. That is because when they are a sign of cleverness rather than simply being weak, such characters are peripheral to the main plotline. After all, glasses are not in the man of action's toolkit. Glasses may befit the proxy to the man of action—the puppet master as with an espionage boss—but here the exceptions only tend to prove the rule. If there is a cohort, a special task force, glasses would be out of place for anyone but the computer hacker-information analyst type. Historically, casting wearers of glasses as secondary characters is deeply entrenched. In religious paintings from the Renaissance onward, they are worn by apostles or church leaders, but never the saints because they have divine powers (all this despite their lives predating glasses, but we've covered that). The biggest contender for glasses, St Jerome, is never depicted with them, but at best with a weary squint. Money-handlers and the like such as merchants and money-lenders are occasionally seen in paintings wearing glasses but once again, these are hardly the sexiest members of the story.

Yet they can be the more compelling. In films where groups consist of types—the fool, the lothario, the sports star, the good kid—glasses confirm the stereotype if not for the social outcast, then for having brains. This is repeated to the point of liturgical conformity in Hollywood feature films and elsewhere. In the 1985 teen flick *The Breakfast Club*, the academically gifted Brian Johnson (Anthony Michael Hall) is distinguished by the thick rims of his glasses. There are at least three boys with glasses in *Dead Poets Society* (1989), although not the main character (Ethan Hawke) lest he be unappealing. In *Good Will Hunting* (1997), Robin Williams is a psychologist who presides over the eponymous mathematical prodigy (Matt Damon). He wears a set of rimless specs but curiously, or predictably enough, not on the promotional poster.

The most famous of all characters of recent times is Harry Potter. I will now use that hackneyed and often misused, and now cringeworthy word: iconic. He fits the definition and updates it. An icon is normally religious and involves an instantly recognizable symbol that elicits admiration and respect. An attendant definition relates to ancient Greek statuary of victorious athletes in conventional triumphal poses. This also works because even for those who have only fleeting exposure to the books, the illustrations, and the movies, the image is always of Harry Potter as bright-eyed behind his glasses, intent, alert, becloaked, brandishing a wand. Harry Potter is the ultimate earnest deliverer of benign retribution. He even has a spell that immediately mends his glasses when they are smashed, quite a quaint antiquarian touch not out of alignment with others, yet in reality his lenses would most likely have been plastic, but to have them so would have missed a dramatic possibility.

It is impossible to name a reliable statistic, but there is enough anecdotal evidence, coupled with the knowledge of how fandom figures influence action and appearance, that Harry Potter steered glasses, and his kind of frames in particular, to become chic. Concomitantly, the tie to nerdiness was brought down a few notches on the negative scale. The Harry Potter phenomenon began in 1997 with the first novel, *Harry Potter and the Philosopher's Stone* followed by six more, with the first film released in 2001. This was precisely at a time when cosplaying—communities right up to conventions—was becoming a popular practice for the youth of the day, and where "fandom studies" were emerging as a serious critical pursuit. Cosplayers (and their significant offshoots, Lolitas, who insisted they weren't cosplaying but doing something unique to themselves), introduced a new kind of dressing up. While similar, cosplaying was different from Halloween and dressing-up parties, and it was a far more amplified kind of following a trend, as men did by wearing "Brando jackets" following the film *The Wild One* (1953). Cosplaying is more earnestly stepping into the role, personalizing it by a receptive channeling which, depending on the wearer, has strong consequences for shaping and creating identity. In this vein, a wearer of the black, rounded frames with the hinges to the arms at the center rather than the top of the lenses is playing at being Harry Potter. On an everyday level, even if not part of the cosplaying effort, in actively selecting frames resembling Harry's, the wearer participates in all the fantasy, glory, and fun of the popular narrative.

Harry Potter did more than any other fictional character to usher in the new fashion of "geek chic." The website from the specialist fantasy emporium "Ancient Warrior" has this to say:

> In recent years, "geek chic" has become a fashion movement in its own right. What was once considered nerdy is now cool and mainstream. The round frames worn by Harry Potter fit perfectly into this trend. They convey intelligence, creativity, and a sense of individuality.[5]

Popular culture's biggest asset is its permeability through dissemination and repetition, to the extent of taking something normal to the point of habitual. The most salient example of this is Leonardo da Vinci's *Mona Lisa,* which has been rendered all but invisible through its ubiquity. It is routinely consigned to the mythic status of the greatest work of art ever produced, an absurd notion but one that draws a lot of satisfaction. Likewise, Harry Potter, seen on bedside tables, in bookstores, on film posters, in games, in film shorts, in endless advertising incarnations, has seeped deeply into the public consciousness internationally to make glasses a different grade of exceptional. As a youth wearing glasses, you'd have been the exception, while the connotation that this is because of a physical imperfection has shifted to that of having insight and a high level of competence.

Pre-Potter, a short roll call of examples in popular culture are perpetuations of the connection between the brainy and the purblind. Among the Smurfs, created by the Belgian artist who went by the name of Peyo, the character with glasses—formerly *schtroumpf à la lunettes* or glasses-smurf, evolved in English into Brainy Smurf—is more the enactment of smarts, being inclined to unsolicited sententious pronouncements. Also Belgian, the great Hergé, creator of *The Adventures of Tintin* series that did more than anything to usher in the graphic novel as a serious genre, has the recurring character Professor Calculus. Calculus is a physicist and inventor who is also deaf, and his brilliance is comically offset by his lack of dexterity. In all, he is the embodiment to the point of archetype of the absent-minded professor and mad scientist. Then of course there's the inimitable Marcie in Charles

Schulz's *Peanuts*. Marcie is the intellectual of the group. She is the bane of Snoopy's and Charlie Brown's life because of her incisively unwelcome truths. It is all at a cost, which hinges upon the glasses, for not only is she inept at sports but unlucky in love, as she pines for the musical genius Schroeder. Daniel Clowes in *Ghost World* would present a more updated Marcie with his character Enid. In the 2001 film, she is played by Thora Birch and is almost classy with her thick dark glasses, moon face, and rounded black bob and side hairpin. In the comic, she is a great deal grungier and even more prickly, being the mouthpiece for Clowes himself. Her glasses signal her as a person of insight and the part they play in diminished attractiveness is more a liberation because they are a sign that she won't play any part in the love game.

Despite, or maybe because of, the pleasing air of positivity that Harry Potter helped to breathe into the world of glasses, there is still a noticeable dearth of examples in animated series, and they generally veer toward the accepted orthodoxy of what glasses denote (intellect over attractiveness). For the children's films in recent times, Pixar is a good place to start. Scanning the films since *Toy Story* (1995), I can so far find only two instances of glasses. Granted that bugs and monsters don't wear glasses, but who's to say in the fantasy-verse? Fish wearing glasses (*Finding Nemo*, *Finding Dory*) might not be a bad touch because of its self-evident implausibility. The only two seem to be *Inside Out* (2015 and its 2024 sequel) and *Turning Red* (2022), in which glasses are worn by the canny best friend. The former hinges on the externalization of emotions into embodied forms, much as the Mr. Men series (Mr. Clever and, interestingly, Mr. Brave wear glasses) did in the previous century. The personification of sadness is a short, plump girl with blue skin and prominent black circular glasses. While this perpetuates the stereotype of the outcast, there is also that of the smarter: the mother wears glasses, as do all five women at the control panel within her mind. The father's control panel do not, and they are markedly more clueless. But the count stops there, suggesting that the mainstreaming of glasses, however common they may be as items in everyday life, is still selective and still freighted with narrative expectation.

Glasses and youth mean being pinned down to a less wild, more domestic existence, but once the child becomes an adult it is as if all those years of privation and curtailment have borne fruit. So the cliché goes—but as I have hopefully shown already, it is a cliché that has been shaped by fact combined with relentless historical topologizing. People in public office wearing glasses have the air that they are uncaring of the vanities of appearance and that they have led an honest life of study and reflection. Popular wisdom has it that politicians wearing glasses are thought to be more trustworthy than those without them; the wearer sees better, knows better. Donald Trump, who has taken Alpha male bullish virility to a new level of absurdity, is seldom seen wearing glasses, using them only on the rare occasions when he reads. Arguably the first politician, discounting

Franklin, to have given spectacles mainstream respectability is Theodore Roosevelt. Roosevelt was a startlingly agile and voracious intellect coupled with a capacious memory. He was also an intrepid hiker, horse rider, and boxer (which blinded him in one eye), and his contributions to founding national parks associate him intimately with the outdoors. This meant that the glasses were not an impediment so much as an enhancement. This august tradition took a sharp turn for the worse with the advent of Sarah Palin, for whom any sign of sharpness was swiftly undermined by a show of bathos (thanks also to Tina Fey): a person who looks smart but is not presents a possibility ripe for satire.

What if the precarious social approval that young people wearing glasses experience is not tied to conventions of attractiveness? Not limited to narratives of being physically inferior and confined to a protected life without risk or danger? Boring and dowdy in other words. Maybe the analogy is more sinister and is based on a truth that is embarrassing and best left hidden. Let us begin again with glasses and intelligence: glasses are not the master signifier but rather lead one much closer to that conclusion. To reiterate: anyone wearing glasses can be suspected of being smart. It's an easy indicator which we can then test out, but then some recoil because the test might yield grim results.

Arthur Schopenhauer, in section thirty-four of his *Counsels and Maxims*, asserts that on the whole society shrinks from intelligent people because of the base fear of exposure as inferior. "To show your intelligence and discernment," he writes,

> is only an indirect way of reproaching other people for being dull and incapable. And besides, it is natural for a vulgar man to be violently agitated by the sight of opposition in any form; and in this case envy comes in as the secret cause of his hostility. For it is a matter of daily observation that people take the greatest pleasure in that which satisfied their vanity; and vanity cannot be satisfied without comparison to others. Now, there is nothing of which a man is prouder of than of intellectual ability, for it is this that gives him his commanding place in the animal world. It is an exceedingly rash thing to let anyone see that you are decidedly superior to him in this respect, and to let other people see it too; because he will then thirst for vengeance, and generally look about for an opportunity of taking it by means of insult, because this is to pass from the sphere of *intellect* to that of *will*—and there all are on an equal footing as regards the feeling of hostility.[6]

Smart people are routinely ostracized and bracketed because they introduce a level of reality that the more mediocre would prefer hidden. Glasses court this prejudice and spark a primitive reflex. There is a lot in this for the longtime glasses-wearer: as a child it is the sudden and unprovoked insult and the feeling of being kept down to size. And if you *are* smart then you may be relegated to a periphery where your pronouncements are taken not as insight but as risible eccentricity. Being friendly with glass-eyed kids? Risky. Schopenhauer, maybe a little histrionically, mentions the "bitterest feelings of sullen and rancorous hatred" which Nietzsche more temperately translated into the "pathos of distance."

Then the glass-eyed kid becomes an adult. Eyes may have improved, or there is the option of contact lenses. Or glasses have become part of one's person, become more talisman than burden. The pathos of distance engenders a craving for love, or it may find itself in ironic detachment, the glasses a vital, sometimes melancholic, membrane between self and world.

3 LOOKING GOOD

When did glasses become more fashion than function? Maybe it was in the early 1970s, with the late Elvis and John Lennon. It started with men, but this has changed, although there are significantly fewer women who have not built their image around glasses as opposed to sunglasses. Spike Lee, Elton John, and Bono number among the many celebrities who wear glasses informally or where glasses are indelible to their image. When female celebrities do wear them (Jennifer Garner, Anne Hathaway), it is a staged contradiction of covering or mitigating "natural" beauty with the result of reasserting it. It is also the premium placed on female beauty that makes sunglasses so alluring for them, for it is about covering the dazzling prize until it's unveiled to the initiated. Audrey Hepburn's dark glasses in *Breakfast at Tiffany's* (1961) are the strategic accent of elegance to her black dress. Sunglasses are the epitome of cool from Jackie Onassis to the *Men in Black* film franchise to Gangsta fashion. They were the archetypal shield between self and world. When sunglasses are used gratuitously indoors, belying their ordinary function to protect against the sun, they add distinction but usually to the already distinct, otherwise you are a try-hard loser. I'm unaware of anyone in my own life who wears frames with neutral lenses, but that's obviously the point, and most likely the old prejudice kicks in: I overestimate their cleverness.

> I can see you, your brown skin shining in the sun
> You've got your hair slicked back and those Wayfarers
>   on, baby
> I can tell you, my love for you will still be strong
> After the boys of summer have gone

There ends Don Henley's 1984 hit "Boys of Summer." The image is vivid, and so very eighties. It wouldn't be hard to surmise that Henley may have been thinking, consciously or unconsciously, of Tom Cruise in *Risky Business* the year before. The promotional poster is a close-up of his upper face with his eyes staring over a pronounced pair of what are unmistakably black Wayfarers. This was not the first major manifestation of them; they were part of the unmistakable uniform of the 1980 cult film *The Blues Brothers*. In 1986 they would feature again in *Ferris Bueller's Day Off* with Matthew Broderick wearing them with a less lascivious expression that hearkened unmistakably back to Cruise. Meanwhile in that year Cruise assisted yet again in Ray-Ban's corporate fortunes by making their Aviators another staple item. As a classic the Wayfarer is the default style, to sunglasses what Levis 501s are to jeans and white Converses are to sneakers.

That was the main point of the opening scene of Quentin Tarantino's first film *Reservoir Dogs* (1992), which has its biggest stake in sunglasses, and of the Ray-Ban brand especially. Here they are all walking in unison in slo-mo wearing black suits and ties and dark glasses. Three wear Wayfarers, while Mr. Brown (Tarantino) has a pair of Predators (a more feline wraparound style), and Mr. Orange (Tim Roth) has 3016 Clubmasters (a retro style similar in silhouette to the Wayfarer but where the more pronounced part of the frame on the upper rims). While the strong, repeated contrasts make for a graphic visual that is difficult to forget, the sunglasses are what bind them as criminals, and when they come off, they each unravel in all their naked humanity.

Even allowing for *The Blues Brothers* and Tarantino's film, in terms of blockbuster credentials the *Matrix* franchise steals all sunglass glory. The promotional poster for the first in the series (1999) leaves no ambiguity that the cyberpunk shades are indissociable parts of the personae of the main characters, with Neo (Keanu Reeves) at the helm. While hundreds of dark glasses feature throughout the film, his are a special statement that are black, sleek, rimless tapering ovals. Alas, they were custom-made for the film (designed by Richard Walker of Blinde Design Project), but approximations may be found in the Silhouette line. Since they are so prominent throughout the film, sunglasses have a symbolic resonance that chimes with the premise of the entire series, namely that the world that is considered reality is a computer-generated fiction. They keep the wearers slightly disjunct from the deceptive world of appearances while also turning them into ciphers, generic beings, products of a hyper-rationalized system (the Matrix) that is mistaken for reality. For Neo and company they also become standard issue, since he himself did not wear them until he knew he was going to be in the fight for truth, presumably that day when the eyes can roam free. Helping to hide affect, his sunglasses visually certify that he has signed up for official cosmic business together with his cyberpunk-glass-wearing brethren.

Commenting in the wake of the final film in the series, *The Matrix Resurrections* (2021), *The Chicago Tribune* stated that of all the films known for their sunglasses, in the Matrix films they play "the most duplicitous role of all." Fashion curator Kevin Jones contends that: "In just about any film, when you see a person driving a car, they take the rearview mirror away. But here are these sunglasses acting as a rearview mirror so you know what's going on behind you as well as in front of you."[1] They are constant reminders that in the Matrix appearances are manifold and malleable.

Cool and sunglasses conjoin when they are superfluous, as in the Corey Hart one-hit wonder, "Sunglasses at Night" (1984) with the record cover of him in a pair of dark shades, of course. Sunglasses indoors are for the starlet who wants the attention for not wanting the attention. They have long been a useful tool for anyone who is susceptible to too much attention, for celebrities who are liable to have any reaction taken as a sign of something and exaggerated out of proportion. Or they can be used by gangsters and seedy underworld figures. Either way, by covering the eyes you are blocking affect and detaching from the world. There is a certain luxury in doing this, or necessity: the boss with his bodyguards. Dark glasses such as these are also used as a device appreciably dominant in thriller films to create a form of disguise or to generate unease. Whether the wearer can see or not, this artificial barrier suggests a clear (if obscured) difference between them and us. Conventionally—and for most of us who don't hang out in the underworld, we can only draw on film and television—the rest of the company is expected to show themselves as they are, as to do otherwise would be an affront, a challenge to authority and overall just an unwise move because it is a sign that you have some kind of symbolic booty to hide.

There is a telling irony between the organic unity of sunglasses and cool that we tend to take for granted, which is that they hide infirmity and weakness in equal measure with power and beauty and sometimes combine the two. In recent memory, someone who comes briskly to mind is Bono, the lead singer from U2. While he made good use of them in his performances such as in the song "The Fly" where he sported large, hugging, goggle-like black sunglasses, with obvious references, he began wearing tinted glasses in the 1990s because of his battle with glaucoma, a condition of the optic nerve and fluid buildup whose symptoms include photosensitivity. Subject to bright lights and paparazzi camera flashes, without them his right eye swells up. In Bono's words, "it's part vanity, it's part privacy and part sensitivity."[2] The psychological assurance of having a filter from the pell-mell of the outside world can have just as much utility as a prophylactic.

Disregarding the copious recourse to poetic license, one of the reasons that makes the Vernon Fell character so compelling is that anyone with a taste for costume dramas and historical dress-ups would not find it hard to imagine a nineteenth-century dandy or some Victorian rake wearing tinted lenses. In that time, because they were still a rarity, they would have something sinister about them. This is why in Coppola's *Bram Stoker's Dracula* (1992), the Count in his human form when he arrives in London scouring for Mina Harker peers through a blue-tinted pince-nez, a concession to the lethal light sensitivity of vampires which this rendition has conveniently dodged. Dracula (Gary Oldman) is now a mercurial dandy in an impeccable three-piece gray suit, matching top hat, and long curled locks, so very different from the rest of the men in the street, so very "Hungarian." Disguise and affectation, his blue lorgnette is not only an open indicator of his (mortal) foreignness, but also the aloofness afforded by inhuman power. He is in the minority, if not unique, and his sunglasses single him out through the mechanism of his concealment.

How much did the costume designer want us to read into Dracula's pseudo disguise? In the nineteenth century, a certain kind of scissor-action lorgnette was known as the "Parisienne" because they were used by Parisian dandies to eye off passersby with theatrical disapproval. More appropriately, given that Dracula is associated with the pestilence of rats, darkened glasses—not blue but amber yellow or brown—were used in the nineteenth century by sufferers of syphilis whose many symptoms included light sensitivity and subsequently blindness, and worst of all, the eyes falling out of their sockets.

Despite the discovery of the dangers of ultraviolet rays in the 1870s, it would take until the early twentieth century for UV-protecting glasses to be introduced (the first UV-protecting lenses were introduced in 1899). This means that when Dracula crawled the earth at the time of Bram Stoker's tale (1897), the tinted glasses that Dracula would have been wearing (apt to his fastidious taste while in mortal form) would have been from the Venetian Murano glassworks. Since at least the mid-eighteenth century, the Venetians had been relieving their eyes from the dazzling glint of the sun off the water with colored glasses. One beautiful artifact exists that was in the safekeeping of Doge Alvise Giovanni Mocenigo who governed Venice from 1763 until the end of 1778. These were a lorgnette-style face with arms of temple-pieces which were elongated loops as opposed to hooks to secure on the ears. The lenses are an emerald green and for added protection are silk side-guards. The style came to be known as "Goldini" glasses after the Venetian playwright Carlo Goldini who wore them about town as a personal signature.

For women of station as they glided down the canals, the Venetians had invented a paddle holding an elliptical green glass pane, something between a Chinese fan and an enlarged monocle, having a hook that could allow it to hang from the neck, which were known as *vetri da gondola*, "gondola glasses," or *vetri da dama*, "ladies' glasses."[3] In keeping with their resemblance to flat fans, their lacquered surfaces were decorated with Chinoiserie motifs, which in Venice at the time would have been wholly *de rigueur*. It is easy to imagine a stately countess, her governess, and her brood of children on a gondola, the water sparkling and the entire cohort covering their faces with these tinted shields, the children with customized junior-sized ones. The utility of these items could swiftly become misconstrued to seem as keeping their noble station at a distance from unworthy public exposure or commoner's eyes. In the early days when sunglasses were merely tinted lenses, there had always been this accompanying sense of the wearer being at one or two degrees of remove from the hoi polloi.

The green tint of the gondola glasses brings us back to Nero's *smaragdus*, the emerald stone he is reported to have used while watching the carnage in the Colosseum. Perhaps it wasn't that he was shortsighted but that it simply tinted the view and relieved his eyes from the bright sun. So contends the German mid-eighteenth-century writer Lessing in his *Forty-fifth Letter*, a remark that is more telling for the degree of attention devoted to an incidental detail.[4] Given that sight is the most developed sense in humans, it speaks as much to how we have so willingly entertained possibilities of embellishing or varying our vision, and have freely adopted possibilities for visual play. To accept this notion is also to concede that the lenses we hold before our eyes can as much be for palliating or altering the world as to see it with greater accuracy.

When properly protective sunglasses did arrive on the market in the 1930s, the slang in America for them was "sun cheaters" or just "cheaters." I vaguely remember this word still being used in the 1970s, but no longer. It is one of those telling epithets that started out with what was most likely a wholesome cleverness eventuating into something more disturbing and clandestine since sunglasses would be part of the expected uniform for gangsters and card sharks alike. "Sun cheaters" is a far more innocent term since it is not who you are cheating but what—ultraviolet radiation. "Cheaters" is far more paramount and a great deal more apt since sunglasses in effect cheat the onlooker out of knowing what you really look like. Your identity is hidden, but not quite—sunglasses are that gesture that signals that you don't want to give it all up.

Sunglasses are the industrialized veil. When Sam Foster introduced celluloid lenses in 1929, sunglasses became available to everyone. Under the brand name Foster Grant, he set himself up with a stand on the boardwalks of Atlantic City and New Jersey, and in only a decade they were a standard accessory worn well beyond reasons of utility. In 1938, *Life* magazine ran an article with the title "Dark Glasses are New Fad for Wear on City Streets": "For years Hollywood stars have worn dark glasses to protect their eyes from the harmful glare of klieg lights, and to conceal their identity from curious fans. Now dark glasses have become a favorite affectation of thousands of women all over the U.S." It suggests the sale of over twenty million of them the year before but "[o]f the millions that wear them about 25% percent really need them."[5] Where these statistics come from is not disclosed, but the main point is driven home regardless, namely that it speaks to how quickly dark glasses were embraced, and have continued to be so into our own time. The focus on women is not only because they were the natural target of fashion consumption at the time but no doubt also that they were a convenient shield from the prying eyes of men, which of course only rendered them more desirable. Remember that this was when it was not abnormal for men to leer and cat-call. The closing caption reads: "Colored rims to complement faces, or to match frocks and accessories were introduced four years ago in New York. The fad spread quickly."[6]

Now, sunglasses are a huge business and vie with the fragrance industry for the most consumed designer items, and, like perfume, they accompany an embarrassingly wide profit margin. (All the lower-end fragrances are almost entirely synthetics, while sunglasses involve a little metal and are almost entirely plastic.) There is no serious major brand that is without its own line of sunglasses. As with perfume, sunglasses are a way of participating in high-end brand culture with proportionate ease, as their prices do not compare to those of handbags, shoes, watches, or clothing. Where they have it over perfume is that the brand is easily visible even to the point of being a patent advertisement worn over the face. Prada gets away with this tastefully, while Versace all but gives up on discretion because it is grounded in ostentation, a sort of vulgarity that is so brazen that it almost turns a corner back toward being classy. In 2024, the international revenue for sunglasses was over twenty-five billion with almost a billion pieces projected for production by 2029 where profits will be over thirty-five billion.[7]

Tom Ford, who now has a large share of both the perfume and sunglasses markets, comes to the business with his own look in both glasses and sunglasses, usually in a largish, slumped, and rounded aviator style. These add to his image as a man of indomitable sophistication and as someone who knows how to dress, how to dress others, and how to make business flourish (he also directed two very good feature films). There is a promotional picture of Ford, in a slim-fit, black-velvet tuxedo wearing brown-tinted glasses, and behind him is his female counterpart in unimpeachable chic, Anna Wintour, in black glasses (we can only assume Tom Ford's), the paragon of inscrutability. An excerpt from the rather relentless promotional blurb reads:

> Seductive and provocative, the Tom Ford sunglasses are for men and women who are confident and are not afraid to show their sensuous sides. Find your inner *femme fatale* in the form of an oversized, cat-eye frame or let your macho side shine through in pair of aviator shape frames.[8]

Before you collapse from exhaustion you are also reminded that his shades are worn by a myriad of top-list celebrities including Scarlett Johansson, Rita Ora, Eva Longoria, Brad Pitt, Miley Cyrus, Ryan Reynolds, Jennifer Lawrence, Angelina Jolie, Gwen Stefani, and Kate Upton (not necessarily in that order). As if to assuage any doubt as to the fashionable supremacy of the Tom Ford brand, we are reminded that they were worn by Daniel Craig as James Bond in *Skyfall* (2012) and *Spectre* (2015). Evidently there has never been a greater incentive to invest in a pair of the appropriate aviators.

From a cinematic perspective at least, spies as well as confidence tricksters would be incomplete without sunglasses as they serve the dual purpose of accenting the already slick while being a casual disguise. The promotional poster for the comedy thriller *Focus* (2015) has Will Smith and Margot Robbie looking askance and impressive in their sunnies. Without the pop-philosophical flavor of the Matrix, the film is replete with sunglasses for men and women. It does not take a scholar of cinema to ascertain their role as a narrative device, beginning with the title. Nicky is a con man and Jess is a grifter who have a relationship, fall apart, then resume after a few years, and find themselves in trouble because of a lack of "focus."

It is not hard for these film stars to look good in any glasses, but for others, they are a salutary necessity to cover up injury or disfigurement. Battered wives are inclined to sunglasses to avoid attention in public, or they may come in handy for bloodshot eyes after a busy and festive night, or due to a pesky eye infection (stye). They may cover more permanent deformities such as exophthalmos (also called proptosis or exorbitism), which is the chronic bulging of the eyes from the socket. This condition has a large list of known causes, and its effects can be particularly nasty, especially given that the bug-eyed phenomenon can make the afflicted look moronic and monstrous, which means that dark glasses are welcome to all involved. Apparently, this affliction is particularly common in dogs, especially the pug-nosed varieties because of their shallow orbit (the anatomic term for the socket in the skull housing the eye). I wonder if there is a small fortune to be made for canine dark glasses. If they did catch on, they would most likely be worn in the majority by the healthy, given the extent to which many owners are fond of narcissistically projecting themselves onto their pets.

4 LOOKING DIFFERENT

I would wager that even with the many changes in today's popular imagination, if you asked, "Who is the most famous character in history to wear glasses as a disguise?" the answer would still be Superman as Clark Kent. Why this happens to be the case is attributable to two things. One is that he was the first figure in popular culture who had a dual identity that did not involve a mask, and where the whole narrative premise hinged on these two personae. The other is the patent absurdity of it all. How could someone with that height, physique, and those chiseled features hide who he was through a large pair of glasses and some bumbling affectations? The arguments for the disguise working are that Superman is not only physically masked but behaves differently as well. As Christopher Reeve played him in the first major feature films that began in 1978, he is overly loquacious, insecure, positively geeky. But still . . .

The implausibility of Superman's disguise reminds me of one of the funniest clean jokes I know:

Q: What did the man say when he saw three elephants coming over the hill?
A: I don't know.
Q: "There are three elephants coming over the hill." What did the man say when he saw three elephants wearing sunglasses coming over the hill?
A: "There are three elephants wearing sunglasses coming over the hill?"
Q: No, nothing, he didn't recognize them.

While the comic universe may allow for all of this because it is drawn, not photographed, and as such is abstracted and fantasy from the outset, when transposed onto film the conceit is flimsier still. If we skip the television series and the animated shorts of the 1940s and go straight to the first film adaptation of 1978, the need for thick suspension of disbelief is left to the comic fan die-hards who take it all as rote and attribute the same implausibility of his being able to disguise himself to that of having superpowers. In a world where a man can be made of steel and fly, the inhabitants are blissfully bereft of basic empirical deduction when it comes to sizing up other people. This is as much for Reeves in the original as for Brandon Routh and Henry Cavill in the more recent films. The glasses become more than glasses as such but act as a symbolic key or switch from Kent to Superman and back again.

The history of disguise, from at least the perspective of pulp novels, noir, and B-grade films and comics, is one of hiding behind glasses. The humor of the Superman-Kent dynamic lies in the sheer flimsiness of the disguise. It is worth pondering this paradigm for a moment by beginning with the notion that our acceptance of it is something more than a simple suspension of disbelief. It could have to do with the inground prejudice of so many people about the inverse proportion of glasses and physical prowess. Someone as mighty as Superman is so divorced from the glass-eyed nerd that any kind of association is simply not to be entertained. Then again, it could be that his eyesight is so well attuned and superhuman that he needs an extra mitigating layer.

Now we are in X-men territory, with the mutant Cyclops aka Scott Summers who emits beams of energy from his eyes, only held in check by a special eye piece. Those who aren't devotees may need reminding that Superman also has the power of heat vision. Apparently, as the story goes according to the comics, this was harder to control in his youth, especially when he was excitable and his eyes would sort of ejaculate fire spurts. This is what occurred when his friend in high school, Lana Lang, gave him a kiss and he blasted a banner and triggered the sprinkler system. The solution was proposed by his adoptive mother, Martha Kent, to fashion glasses from the alien crystals remaining in the rocket ship that brought him to earth. These would act as an effective barrier until he could get his superpower under control.[1] While this may seem like comic-book trivia, the anecdote reveals a broader cultural idea: glasses as tools for taming youthful excess. They are a mechanism for quelling desire, keeping over-activity in check.

For another reason why Superman was able to keep himself hidden behind Clark, you will have to delve back into the origin story of the comic itself by Jerry Siegel and Joe Shuster, who published the first strip of the Man of Steel in *Action Comics #1* in June 1938. Here the beginning focuses on the cape crusader's feats of superhuman strength. The first panels involving Clark are solely of him poring over the newspapers to ensure that stories about Superman are not there. It also helps that, as a reporter, his current brief is to cover stories on the superhero, which means that he is in an optimal position to vet content. As an affecting bespectacled bumbling maladroit, as Siegel and Shuster admitted on Superman's fiftieth anniversary, he was inspired after Harold Lloyd whose alter ego, Lonesome Luke, appeared in 1915. He was a complete rivalrous knock-off of Charlie Chaplin's tramp and while Chaplin was still recognized as the premier comedian, Lloyd was a fierce challenger who made more money because he made more films. Lloyd then decided to do more than just imitate and branch out on his own with his own characters resulting in "Glass," otherwise called "The Boy." Lonesome Luke was left behind as a lovable dunderhead with glasses.[2]

Lloyd would later state that the glasses, which were very much a rarity in film and in popular culture of the time, were a masterstroke because they humanized him:

> When I adopted the glasses, it more or less put me in a different category because I became a human being. He was a kid that you would meet next door, across the street, but at the same time I could still do all the crazy things that we did before, but you believed them. They were natural and the romance could be believable.[3]

But that was happenstance, and not the motivation for them. They in fact came to be worn due to the old chestnut of glasses decreasing attractiveness. Hal Roach, who produced Lloyd's early films (as he would the Laurel and Hardy series), thought him too handsome to sustain the kind of familiar slapstick that would endear him to his audience. They were not only to distance him from Lonesome Luke, but to turn him into the most unlikely (and therefore memorable) fellow to occupy a silver screen. So, in creating Clark Kent, Siegel and Shuster were drawn to the ungainliness of Lloyd's character and also that he had disguised himself away from the persona he had previously played.[4]

However, contrary to what common sense may seem to dictate, there is wisdom to suggest that Superman's disguise may indeed work. Glasses are, after all, no longer permitted on identity cards or passports. Research carried out at the University of Kent in the mid-2010s found that people did not easily draw connections between the same person with and without glasses. Then psychologists for this study showed the participants several informal, as opposed to passport-like, photographs like those found on social media. These were then shown in pairs according to the three possible permutations: both glasses, both without, or with and without. In asking whether they could see that it was the same person or not, the first two categories drew the greatest accuracy of about eighty percent, while the last had an accuracy rate of around 74 percent.[5]

One of the scientists, Robin Kramer, asserted that a key factor in being able to deduce the same face was familiarity. "When a security guard checks a passport photo against the person standing in front of them, they do not have the luxury of familiarity with that face, as Lois does with Superman/ Clark Kent." Lois would have no trouble in deducing Superman's true identity, but as co-worker Kay Ritchie avers, "For those who do not know him, however, this task is much more difficult, and our results show that glasses do disrupt our ability to recognize the same unfamiliar person from photo to photo."[6] We have an intuitive awareness of this already, drawn from casual experience. Wearing glasses, while not a wholesale transformation, does disrupt a habitual association of the naked face, which is also why still in so many narratives and films they are a finishing touch to anyone escaping an adversary or going undercover.

In the celebrity department, as part of "looking good," the transformation that glasses bring is a cap on getting older. Spectacles offer an easier, slow transition for fans of those they presume to be genetically blessed and immune to old age. For the celebrity, it is a demonstration that they have accepted the next stage in their life and that they are embracing age with a degree of grace. Or that they are confident that their charisma and good looks can withstand almost anything.

Beyond the Superman paradigm, the ultimate glasses disguise is the glasses modeled off Groucho Marx's appearance, hence "Groucho glasses." These are black round frames affixed with a large plastic nose, a bushy black mustache, and equally bushy eyebrows stuck to the top of the frames. Sold as early as the 1940s, these are the most widely recognized novelty. Lawrence Bush adds:

> The stereotyped Jew, on the other hand, being associated with money and business, was less comical and therefore less likely to appear . . . Sam Oumano's Franco-American Novelty Company nevertheless found the "fun" in Jewish stereotyping when it produced "Beagle Puss" in the 1970s, popularly called "Groucho Marx glasses" (with an oversized plastic nose and shaggy mustache and eyebrows), advertised as "The World's Funniest Disguise . . . Make fun of city slickers!"[7]

Whether or not this item carries the stigma of anti-Semitism is a matter of taste as they are now the most generic of mock disguises, and the first go-to for those who still know who Groucho Marx was and just want to channel his buffoonery.

Groucho is one of those people in popular memory who is inseparable from their glasses. But unlike the product named after him, the spectacles he wore were more frequently steel-rimmed. The glasses are the beginning of his comic *accoutrements*, continuing with his exaggerated greasepaint mustache and, of course, the cigar. To remove the glasses and the rest of the ensemble would be an emasculation, a neutering of his essential self; Groucho dressed up as Groucho but without the costume there is nothing left. In more obvious dress-up and for comic effect is Barry Humphries' alter ego Dame Edna Everage who, as the character evolved, would wear ever more outrageous frames. These were largely of the cat's-eye variety where the tips were an opportunity for adding sundry extra decoration, such as three or more diamantine tendrils extending upward and outward, or a panoply of stars. Only Elton John—who has worn pink-tinted glasses in the shape of hearts—can rival "her."

Perhaps before Lennon or Elton, the singer who made glasses his indelible mark was the short-lived Buddy Holly. Those big, thick frames would have been noticeable from a considerable distance. They didn't make him look smarter—if anything, they made him seem dopier—but they gave him a wholesome, boy-next-door charm. I cannot find any image of him without them, and no one can fathom one anyway. Unintentionally most likely, John Denver perpetuated the honest as opposed to clever look with his glasses. But while Buddy Holly was like a comic book character that had been brought miraculously to life, Denver's specs always seemed to me incongruous because he was a country and western singer who sang about forests and mountains, the province of Marlboro men without any hint of delicacy. Whereas

Denver's frames are now consigned to obscurity, Buddy's were found months after the plane crash in 1959 where they were taken to the local sheriff until they found their resting place in the Buddy Holly Centre in Lubbock, Texas, his hometown.[8] His glasses were such a visual remnant of who he was, and they were big and are now an artifact.

Choosing the right glasses is a strategic decision—one influenced by shape, size, material, and brand. With celebrities, most likely a stylist is involved. What is key to approaching the appropriate choice of glasses is not to see them as just an extra to the face, an extension of the features. Rather, it is a complement to the face as a foil to the features you have. I know that not everyone is equipped to make such decisions, as the general rule is that we are far better at judging others than ourselves. Strong features may not warrant something light and rimless but may call for reaffirmation with big, bold frames which may also redirect from any facial disproportions.

The standard face taxonomy is a convenient half dozen: round, oval, heart, diamond, square, and pear. It would probably be a slippery slope these days to correlate these roughly to racial groups, so I leave that to the reader's imagination. Round faces are self-explanatory and easy to pick, and the oval is something of the default for facial structure. Heart consists of a pointy chin with a broad forehead. Diamond faces have prominent cheekbones with a tapering chin and small forehead, while square faces have similar proportions between forehead and chin, that's probably Superman with his strong square jaw. The unfortunately named pear shape is someone with a broad jawline but a smaller forehead.

As an example of the offsetting that glasses can perform, cat's-eye glasses are suitable for round faces, which may now send your mind racing to how many chubby women you know who have intuitively chosen the style. Cat's-eyes are a favorite of drag queens irrespective of face shape. They may also be sympathetic to pear and diamond faces because the upward movement counteracts any downward trajectory of the physiognomy. Round glasses are the nemesis of round faces unless you want to court comments behind your back. They counteract angularity so square and rectangular faces and, at a pinch, pear faces. By contrast, round, heart, and oval faces are at their best with rectilinear, square, and oblong glasses, sharp lines mitigating the softer facial contours. Somewhere in the middle are oval glasses which may suit pear faces and be conducive to square and diamond shapes. This is probably too technical, but it is built into the lucrative glasses industry and versions of the above serve as a rubric for run-of-the-mill optometrists so that they can cite an official aesthetic catechism instead of relying on the vagaries of personal taste. Yet in the end, personal taste matters. Angular glasses on an angular face may send a certain signal about a personality, just as round on round may have a festive effect on proud rotundity.

Physiognomics may no longer have the same sinister ring as it once had, for it was previously a pseudoscience used to assign particular traits to races and also to distortions owing to congenital defects. At its most extreme, it was extrapolated to justify certain diagnoses or even eradication. The classifications for face shapes are a much watered-down version of physiognomics and mercifully without the biological baggage. However, that optometrists and sundry glasses brands have gone to such lengths to break down what best serves one kind of physiognomy over another tends to confirm that glasses do have a transformative role to play.

This is why they are almost inevitably in spy and thriller movies. It would be far too tiresome to read out the litany here, but I could zone in on one of the classic thriller films, or as it now transpires, *The Day of the Jackal* based on the book by Frederick Forsyth. This book, and the first adaptation from 1973, were among the first in the thriller genre that spun off the James Bond phenomenon, both in writerly inspiration (after Ian Fleming) and in the resultant films. It is classed as a "political thriller" which we in retrospect can say was the natural by-product of the Cold War. I can still vaguely remember the film at the time and my father's excitement at seeing the film after reading the novel, but I revisited it after having avidly followed the 2024 television series and having enjoyed *The Jackal* from 1997. The latter, starring Richard Gere as the cop and Bruce Willis as the villain (not a hit but still worth seeing) is a smorgasbord of sunglasses and disguises, but the original gives glasses quite a noticeably operative role. (In another Bruce Willis film, the third in the *Die Hard* franchise, the villain played by Jeremy Irons appears in a key scene at the Federal Reserve Bank wearing pert octagonal sunglasses with dark blue lenses which are a dead giveaway that he is not there to make a deposit.)

The original *Jackal* narrative revolves around de Gaulle's granting independence to Algeria in 1962, which incites a failed assassination attempt on him by a dissident group who see the handover as a betrayal of France. Following that, they enlist a crack British killer, the "Jackal," for half a million dollars, an exorbitant sum for that time. Played by the young Edward Fox, the Jackal strikes a dashing figure, always in finely tailored suits, neatly laundered shirts, and often sporting a cravat. The premium on the anti-hero's appearance would be something that the teleseries would emulate, down to the neckerchiefs which, in the present day, mark him out as rather raffish. In the 1997 version, the Jackal is less dapper and instead is a master of disguises, whereas in the first version it is his refusal to hide his appearance that makes the final transformation so much more dramatic. Fleeing the police on the way to Paris, the assassin assumes the identity of an unassuming Danish schoolteacher looking very straight and serious with slicked-back hair and dark, thick-rimmed glasses. In a decisive turning point in the film, as the story builds to its climax, the glasses complete his efforts to alter his appearance, where hitherto no effort had been taken. The glasses in this persona are like a transitional moment, as his final disguise as an aged war veteran is incomplete without them.

This may seem like a minor detail but that's the point—it's small, yet central and consistently used. Glasses are the *sine qua non* of what is brought out at key intervals of dissimulation, betrayal, or concealment in novels and, because they are visible to us, in film. This means that when intentionally placed within the narrative stream they play a structural role that is unlike glasses in real life, let alone when they are worn by celebrities outside of films.

It is then this instrumental, contributing element of glasses to the narrative of the film, to seeing and not being seen, and its role very much as costume as opposed to utility that opens up possibilities for the public image of celebrities wearing them informally, not as actors. When captured wearing them in public, celebrities can not only signal, in the most disingenuous way of course, that they are not guided by vanity and that they just want to get on with living their daily lives. Most crucially, when glasses are worn in public especially by actors cinematically best known to be without them, they register an absence of formality, a sign that cannot be anything but winning. In a way, it is hard for them to lose.

Do not be fooled, though, as glasses worn in this way by well-known and envied people seen otherwise are just another kind of disguise. When so self-consciously bespectacled, they can then play at the private persona, the guise of the undisguised, except that they are an outer layer, symbolic protection. Worn in this way by public figures, glasses have become desirable appendages because of the game of intimacy that they immediately take up, and safe in any accusation of wiliness or self-love because it sets out to espouse the opposite. Any aging actor seen without glasses for any great length of time risks precisely that accusation, sacrificing what is needed and imminent to us all for the sake of image. In sum, for a person whose livelihood is reliant on looks, they are brought into a cryptic or Möbius-strip relation when it comes to glasses. They're no longer just an accessory, but a device that introduces a new kind of play between the confession of age and the benefits of such a confession, of being merely human and being congratulated for being merely so. So endowed, they have that priceless quality which most of them have not earned: *gravitas*. For such people, glasses can be an investment in prejudice: what is for the young and unseen an impediment that consigns them to the margins of heredity is for the hereditarily endowed a virtue that, in the admission of their humanness, keeps them looking down on us with or without a squint.

5 LOOKING INWARD

Wearing sunglasses at night isn't always about projecting allure—it can also signal a deliberate retreat, a symbolic alignment with the visually impaired. For those with sight, to reduce your vision is to reduce what you can do, which places you in a passive role. While sunglasses may tantalizingly cover the bewitchingly beautiful, they are there to save us from uncomeliness as well. They may cover a wandering, lazy, or jerky eye, or worse, no eye at all. They can be the more surreptitious solution to an eye patch in our world that makes you resemble a latter-day pirate, drug lord, or comic-book villain. Glasses can spare the wearer or anyone else the embarrassment caused by seeing eye impairments. Irregularities of the eyes are a special kind of ugliness because they are, as the hackneyed saying goes, the windows to the soul. In sincere conversation, it is eye contact that we seek, as it is there that we get our first impression of a person's demeanor and intentions. Dark glasses are *de rigueur* for funerals and for mourning, as they allow for a brief departure from the rest of the world. In the words of Queen Margaret in Shakespeare's *Henry VI* Part II: "And even with this I lost fair

England's view / And bid mine eyes be packing with my heart / And call'd them blind and dusky spectacles, / For losing ken of Albion's wished coast" (3.2.1754).

One famous person that used dark glasses as a way of retreating while in public spaces was Karl Lagerfeld. Sure, he was a high-end fashion designer and wearing them was not that out of place. But for Lagerfeld, they were far more than that. Bono has his tinted glasses which are not only for his glaucoma but as a mild buffer, wearing dark glasses in unsunny places was a way of accommodating a sensitive, if not fragile soul. Not that he wore them as a signature all the time, although more often in later years. The television series *Becoming Karl Lagerfeld* (2024), with Daniel Brühl in the lead role, beautifully bears this out, showing how the gruff and flamboyant exterior was a mask for extreme vulnerability and a fear of intimate human contact. Emotional turmoil together with exacting standards and a preternatural capacity for work meant that he was destined for loneliness. As well as his rise to fame in the callous halls of haute couture, the series traces the early days of Lagerfeld's longtime companion, Jacques Bascher, the love of his life with whom he nonetheless remained celibate, or so the story goes. For Lagerfeld, who at the height of his fame was barraged with requests and objections (including the old chestnut of the skinniness of models), the dark glasses were a necessary shock absorber. They were also what kept the real Karl from the one that the world wanted to see.

This need to remain within yourself while in public is wholly in keeping with poker players who need dark glasses to retreat into their inner world and to betray no telltale affect. Beyond that of "counting cards"—deducing from the play the likelihood of cards available—poker is a game of feints, bluffs, and "tells." These are all the telltale signs that amount to what the player is thinking and feeling: an inadvertent scratch here, a twitch there, shuffling in the seat, a spontaneous grimace, extra sweating. Some poker purists argue that only amateurs wear dark glasses, while others contend that bodily cues are often involuntary and that they are simply impossible to contain. At least with dark glasses, some of these responses can be averted, from a blink to a twitch, perhaps even a dilated eyeball when dealt a good hand. Protected from the bright lights, they also allow for an uninhibited look at the chips or a glance at your opponent. All the time you are also permitted a quieter, more concentrated absorption.

Mirror glasses have the added advantage of a deflection effect that can distract from any other facial tics, but with the concern that they could reflect your cards; that all depends on where you place them and how you look at them. It may come as no surprise that a company based in New Port Richey in Florida specializes in poker shades. "Blue Shark Optics" has as its by-lines "Because the hunt demands vision: protect your eyes, operate in stealth mode, get clear crisp vision at the tables," and "Dark glasses belong in the sun, not at the poker table." The product icons show the various styles, but with the common denominator of golden lenses, all of which have images of casino halls. No doubt these are geared to dissemble and disconcert.

That there are dedicated products does not necessarily mean that glasses are a fixture in professional poker tournaments. Allegations that wearing sunglasses while playing raises the suspicion of cheating are based on the practice of card-marking specifically to be picked up by specially tinted lenses. Barry Carter, writing on the website PokerStrategy.com, maintains that sunglasses during poker are superfluous and overrated because very few players can read tells at that level of intricacy. Sunglasses themselves are the tell, says Carter, indicating that the wearer is uncomfortable with playing live and that they are genuinely unsociable. The only concession to them might be the distracting degree of bright lights. Where the real problem lies, adds Carter, is where glasses are augmented with purpose-driven, but undetectable technology. The verdict: just as you are no longer allowed to bring in liquids through airport security, so sunglasses of any kind should be banned as a message that cheating in any form is grimly condemned.[1] You must keep your face public. What for most outsiders would first think is a fairly niche concern, covering the eyes is evidently the source of heated debate.

For those of us who take our sight for granted, we become quite uncomfortable when our sight begins to fail, when you have to squint when inspecting products at the supermarket, or when your teenager shows you something funny on his phone and you are forced to admit that you cannot read it because you don't have your glasses at hand, or just having forgotten your glasses and having to strain under a light or use the lamp on your phone. But we can see. Although we become brutally aware that we don't see as well, and we become more sensitive to a sliding scale of satisfactory sight, we still habitually tend toward the binary of sight and non-sight, light and dark. When we see someone with dark glasses and a cane, we assume that she or he is blind, but this is not necessarily true.

What is considered blind, or "legally" blind as it is termed, may still entail a small amount of sight: shadows, dark blurry shapes coalescing into one another, flashes and pulses of gray nebulae. Light sensitivity is different for those with poor vision because the normal recourse to squint can dramatically reduce what can be seen. Beyond utility, wearing dark glasses can signal these limitations from a distance and may also be an aesthetic choice of the wearer. Wearing dark glasses even for those with perfect eyesight is a mild retreat from the world, whereas for those with poor or next to no vision they are a removal from the world many times over. I am sure I am not alone in feeling the chasm between myself and someone known to be blind, enhanced by the glasses. They are the unequivocal register that the person relies on a different sensory logic from ours and configures the world in a different way, the blackness of the glasses a stark reminder of the blackness that engulfs them. It is also to tell us that their differing conjugation of the world means they inhabit a sensory language foreign to ours, and although we would never forego our capacity to see, we are nonetheless curious of this different occupancy of the world and what it may yield to them that it does not ours. Dark glasses might also spare the sighted the unease of not just being unable to look squarely into the eyes, but also perhaps that they, not the blind, are deficient because of a conventional way of apprehending phenomena.

It is no surprise then that many significant figures whom we recall wearing dark glasses are musicians. Music is a form of willful blindness, which is why it is not unusual for people to close their eyes when listening to it, letting their inner eye take over or to extinguish it altogether. For although music may conjure images in some quasi-cinematic way, imaginative projections, or memories, there is also the quality in it that prevails that can dispense with them, where pitch, melody, ambient sound waves, and rhythm stir in a way that no longer requires a referent, unmoored from names and things. In the words of Samuel Beckett, after citing Schopenhauer again, music is "the Idea itself, unaware of the world of phenomena, existing ideally outside the universe, apprehended not in Space but in Time only." This is what makes it "an art that is perfectly intelligible and perfectly inexplicable."[2] This may stir the gentle reader to try a pair of dark glasses when listening to their favorite piece of music.

For starters, try Joaquin Rodrigo's *Concerto de Aranjuez* (1939), one of the most beloved works for guitar in the classical repertoire, then his *Fantasia para un gentilhombre* ("Fantasy for a gentleman"). I have known these pieces since I was about fifteen and listened to them so often that I had to go on a hiatus as it had become so familiar. What I was completely ignorant of was that Rodrigo was blind, having lost it at the age of three from contracting diphtheria. In seeing pictures of him with dark glasses, my obtuse adolescent mind with its undeveloped frontal cortex just assumed that he was a bit of a dude who hung out in the Spanish sun in Valencia. Now knowing otherwise means I cannot listen to his music in the same way.

One of the many appealing elements of the music is that it does not tell you to sit up and listen as, say, a Bruckner symphony does, but it beckons, cajoles, takes you by the hand and asks you to accompany it. Appropriating folk music had been done well before the Romantic composers in the early nineteenth century, and his Aranjuez concerto combines what will seem like familiar excerpts from traditional Spanish guitar themes but meanders in many directions, from the grandiose (those surges in the third movement that put cinema music to shame) to the intimate. Equipped with this new understanding I grasp this piece all the better, as it simulates and transposes a guitarist in a garden together with his own inner emotive stirrings with the sounds of birds and wind, maybe a gramophone in the distance, much as a blind person captures the multiplicity of sounds and thoughts to translate them into a higher sense. Rodrigo described the work as evoking "the fragrance of magnolias, the singing of birds, and the gushing of fountains" in the gardens of Aranjuez.[3]

Rodrigo's insistence on images, smells, sounds, and deep ambience is synesthetic: the correlation of the qualities of one sense with that of another. It is also a real but rare neurological condition caused by the brain routing sensory information of more than one sense. This may give way to words linked to tastes, letters fusing with colors, or sounds brought together with abstract visual data. Although blind, Rodrigo was not unique in his musical intentions, which had been around either since music began in its imitation of birdsong, or more recently when Romanticism sought to strip musical form of its former strictures, placing a premium on the experiential and evocative. Debussy's *Images* (1901–5) is a suite of six piano works that invoke their titles such as "Reflections in the Water," "Bells Through the Leaves," or "Goldfish." To listen to Richard Strauss's *Alpine Symphony* (1915) is to be transported to musical-cinematic vistas but with the images all your own.

Music's call for blindness is not for blackness but for a more profound, inward vividness. This complex and intimate connection is brought out in one of the great and most influential synaesthetic works in the Western musical repertoire: Beethoven's sixth symphony, also called the *Pastoral Symphony* (1808). Its swelling, pulsing passages compel the listener across open fields while the flutes and piccolos mimic the chirping and warbling of birds overhead. It is also the centerpiece for André Gide's 1919 novella of the same name about a pastor and his doomed love for his adopted daughter. Key to his initiation of her into the visible world is Beethoven's symphony, through which he describes a world of shapes and colors. While there is no reference to dark glasses in the book, nor in the film adaptation in 1946, Gide's work does a great deal to demystify the interiorized but sensorily ventilated world of the blind, of which the dark glasses and the raised, undirected head are a powerful and lasting symbol.

In popular music and jazz, the familiar names are Stevie Wonder and Ray Charles, but that shouldn't allow us to forget Diane Schuur or Terri Gibbs. All were born blind or became blind near birth. The exception to those with congenital conditions was Gibbs, whose retinas were damaged from uncovered eyes when she was placed in an incubator after she was born.[4] In 1998, Charles invited Schuur to accompany him, and as she entered, led in by a stagehand, Charles announced that this was "the first time I didn't know what I was doing and they did." Schuur, wearing an oval cat's-eye style pair of dark glasses finished on the outer edges with diamantines, replied: "You look so handsome!" "I know that! [laughter] Thank you, darlin', you're a sweet girl." She settled beside him on a grand piano, and Charles stated to the audience that his "whole purpose is to listen, and I want you to do the same thing, this girl is somethin' else." After "seeing" his hairdo, Schuur sings Isham Jones' 1924 standard, "It Had to Be You," with Charles at his Kurzweil synthesizer.

The footage of this performance defies definition and is worth seeking out.[5] Charles and Schuur sit close to one another, reasonable to say much closer than had they sight, and there is a rapport of energy between them that is palpable. A popular, familiar song, it doesn't demand serious listening, but the presence and actions of the performers have nearly equal importance as the music they make. We see their image and hear their voices and playing, yet their experience is entirely different from ours, built not solely on sounds and rhythm but on the language between themselves generated by the motion of their bodies and the sound waves they emit. Their dark glasses act as containers, as points of concentration and restraint for everything other than sight to issue forth.

In many ways Stevie Wonder (née Stevland Hardaway Morris) brings to popular apogee what Ray Charles put in motion, a blind singer-songwriter-musician equaling any of the sighted. A musical prodigy since a child, it is impossible to gauge to what degree Wonder's impetus and progress were impelled by his inability to see. Happily, in art such things are immeasurable. He has never been shy of being seen with his glasses off, but it is with them on that he is best known. Over a career since the 1960s, he has worn countless kinds of glasses, mostly black, but also occasionally tinted. In a 1981 performance of "Master Blaster" his black glasses had an extra diamantine line between lenses and rims. When he dies, I'll wager there will be a huge exhibit somewhere of all the glasses he had in his possession.

My favorite anecdote about Stevie Wonder is during the recording of "We Are the World" in January 1985, the US response to British 1984 charity hit "Do They Know It's Christmas." Ever wanting to outdo their predecessor, initiators Michael Jackson and Lionel Richie and producer Quincy Jones summoned the Avengers of American pop music at the time. Diana Ross, Bruce Springsteen, Kim Carnes, Ray Charles, Bob Dylan, and of course Wonder were among the twenty-one singers who had solo segments. But Dylan was spooked. Ever the single folk-poet, he may have been used to huge crowds but was completely out of his element with such a concentration of celebrity and hype. In one of the breaks, when his own solo was pending, Wonder took him aside and made a few suggestions about how to sing it. His segment: "There's a choice we're makin', we're saving our own lives, it's true we make a better day just you and me." Then the chorus after which he reprises the last line, and the last words are ineffably Dylan. Wonder apparently counseled him to Dylan-ize them with protracted stress: "just yoooou and meeee." I wonder if a sighted singer would have had the insight or the chutzpah to have done this.

Inspired by such stories, I hope it is not too presumptuous or ignorant for me to add a parable of my own about a fictional blind person. It follows the same lines of fairy tales and real events of people who have suddenly received their heart's desire, usually huge wealth, only to realize that they had been much happier before. Someone blind from birth has known nothing but smell, touch, and sound, and is sensitive to the energies of bodily movements and the smallest changes in the air. All the senses can be brought into powerful harmony but also individually deployed for pleasure or utility.

One day, the person is miraculously granted perfect vision. In ceremony, the dark glasses are removed, and the eyes adjust to the brightness a new complex of the world suddenly comes to light. Not long after, the person feels a stirring in the body, as if it is slowly recalibrating and becoming something else. The sensations of before are less acute, dulled even. The person distrusts this shift in being as those senses had become friends, allies. In response, the glasses are returned, in the case that they are lost, but as if in defiance, the strength and dominating potential of vision vies with the other senses, relentlessly quelling them. The person asks for glasses that are darker and darker until they are opaque and with side-guards to mask any residual light which has become a distraction. This proves better, the senses are happy again and the integrity of the world is restored, for sight had disturbed the balance that had been created between the many stimuli and the closed, private inner world, which was its own sanctuary.

6 LOOKING INTO THE FUTURE

Night glasses, smartglasses, iGlasses—a new generation of eyewear awaits us that mediates between not only our eyes but our eyes and our consciousness. These are the ultimate prostheses that await us in the imminent future, which have already been (imaginarily) demonstrated in thrillers and sci-fi films. They will be devices to unlock the surface of the world, where seeing better is to descry, decrypt, and deconstruct.

The new line of smartglasses by Raty-Ban is called "Meta." It includes an HD camera for photography and video and speakers, what we might already call basic functions when considering the (as yet not rolled out) Apple iGlasses which are expected to interface with your smartphone and watch, producing maps, menus, and icons before your very eyes. But Ray-Ban's choice of the brand name "Meta" is what is most telling: "meta" derives from the Greek for "with, across, or after." It can also mean "outside," as in "metaphysics." I wonder whether this was a conscious decision or just another marketing reflex that places a racy prefix before a commonplace noun.

At the introduction's close I compared the experience of the blind with that of the smartglasses user, where each entailed a complementary embodiment. The former is re-embodiment by necessity, the latter is disembodiment by choice. The smartglasses take you beyond the body and beyond what is immediately seen toward a manifold trans- and metavision. They are not simply an improvement of simple vision but project vision into countless spaces, traversing vast mists of imagery and data. Where once magnifying stones then lenses affixed to the nose were a means of correcting faulty vision, smartglasses (let them be called that from now on) are a different kind of prosthesis in the cyborg vein. To use them is to imply that the sight of the things before us are prosaic givens and need to be surmounted or stripped away, much as our bodies may no longer be the essential mortal core of our being but the mere raw material for shaping and enhancement.

For a few decades now, the talk of the next generation of prostheses has been on having them embedded into the body so that the computers on which we type and tap are incorporated within us. This also means that glasses as we have known them for over seven centuries will become an anachronism. Even dark glasses used for avoiding recognition could scarcely evade sophisticated detection technology made possible by the extra eyes.

"Bionics," the word for the fusion of biology and electronics, has paled since the standardization of chip technology and mostly refers to the more clunky systems that preceded it. Nonetheless, no one of a certain age can forget the *Six Million Dollar Man* and *The Bionic Woman*, who were rebuilt to become Cold-War-warrior super-agents to fight for the (American) good. In today's reckoning, six million dollars does not seem much of an investment in someone destined to save your country many times over, but it was impressive enough in 1973 when the *Six Million Dollar Man* first aired. Who can forget the precredit scene of the show? It begins with emerging as-typed illuminated bluish, heavily pixelated computer text that appears quaint to the contemporary eye: "A C'BORG: A HUMAN BEING WHOSE ORIGINAL HUMAN PARTS HAVE HAD TO BE REPLACED TO ONE EXTENT OR ANOTHER BY MACHINES THAT PERFORM THE SAME FUNCTIONS." And equally quaint to us now is that clarification is needed (the show was based on the 1972 novel *Cyborg* by Martin Caldin). Steve Austin (Lee Majors) is a test pilot flying into space, but the spacecraft is faulty and crashes prematurely. "Steve Austin, astronaut, a man barely alive. Gentleman, we can rebuild him. We have the technology. We have the capability to make the world's first bionic man." At this point is an image of a gridded head schema with an ocular device in the left eye that is linked across the brain to the cerebral cortex. The bionic eye is then shown before it is inserted.

Steve Austin's bionic eye is undetectable (saving money each episode with the make-up department) except when he stops to see things from a telescopic distance unavailable to human capabilities. When this occurs, the camera closes up to Steve's attentive face to a sound that mixes electronica bounce with simulated sonar, the source of countless boyhood simulations across the world for several generations (*mea culpa*).

As with so many of these futuristic conceits and hopeful functions, they are built around some grain of truth. Along with the artificial luxuries of smartglasses for those that already see are glasses that can bring a more qualitative awareness to those that can't. Built into the glasses for the visually challenged can be alerts and cues that warn against obstacles and facilitate more independent decision-making. There are several kinds, including "Envision" and "Invision" versions. Built into the former is an artificial voice system that is a surrogate for reading or identifying documents and such items as banknotes. The wearer/user can also use his or her own voice to make calls. Invision is more of a head device that is controlled by the voice and includes a camera and adjustable magnification that also scans QR and bar codes.

Another recent invention is the ARIA ("Augmented Reality in Audio") glasses for any level of vision impairment that uses[1] sound and sensors to help the user navigate a space. The best way to think of these is as a more sophisticated and personalized model of the sensors built into your car to assist in parking and to avoid collision with nearby objects. One of the inventors, Robert Yearsley, stated in 2023 that: "The glasses are a new form of sensory augmentation that combines elements of visual perception and spatial awareness." Built into the glasses are three tiny video cameras connected to an AI system that uses sound to inform the user about the location of objects in the immediate vicinity. "The speakers," Yearsley continues, "which are located in the arms of the glasses, transmit an intuitive illusion of the location of specific objects which is updated in real time, relative to the user's body and head position." Equipped with such glasses, blind people are considerably relieved of the extra assistance that they require in critical spaces and occasions such as steep, unfamiliar stairs or getting into a taxi. The glasses provide unintrusive sound cues that signal the proximity of nearby objects such that they may be touched, handled, or avoided with a high degree of accuracy, from locating a coffee cup on a bench to differentiating vegetables and fruit in a shop.

Sci-fi punsters among us will cast our minds to the inimitable Geordi La Forge from *Star Trek: The Next Generation* (1987–94), played by LeVar Burton. In the first season, Lieutenant Commander La Forge was helmsman for the USS Enterprise-D, then served as chief engineer. La Forge was blind from birth, requiring him to wear a VISOR before he was given prosthetic implants, "cybernetic eyes," in the later series. VISOR—"Visual Instrument and Sight Organ Replacement"—is like the medieval helmet with an eye-slit, except in reverse, where the slit has materialized around the head. (The term didn't appear in the series proper but only in offshoots such as novelizations.) According to the ordinances of the Star Trek fictional universe, the VISOR is an electromagnetic scanner that, through sensors on the convex side of the fixture, then translates the visual data to the optic nerves and then the brain via the jacks affixed to the temple. Because the VISOR is more like an energy sensor that approximates as opposed to replaces vision, it can detect physiological responses such as pulse, breathing, and bodily temperature, making it a tool in gauging physiological responses such as fear or lying—in humans, but not in aliens.

Although La Forge's apparatus is a constant source of discomfort, during the Star Trek narratives, he has made it his own and is disinclined to separate from it. In the series, he is twice given the chance to dispense with it, but refuses. La Forge's eyepiece is a persistent reminder throughout the series of the conjunction of humans with technological appliances, and that the prosthetic arrangement is not an anthropocentric equation of body plus appendage equals enhanced or corrected body but instead one of symbiosis in which the body can no longer be thought to be the defining element. Instead it is a catalyst for technological interaction.

Night vision glasses, the most modest and commonplace of transformative eye enhancements, are best known to us from thriller movies, or at least those of us who haven't had military training. We associate them with the night-sight headgear from wartime dramas since the post-9/11 incursion in Iraq and Afghanistan, but they have been around for longer than that, now for almost a century. One of the earliest occasions for them was at the hands of a Hungarian physicist based in Britain, Kálmán Tihanyi, who in 1929 devised vision systems as defense against enemy aircraft. This came in the form of a television camera with infrared sensitivities.

Other sources are more liable to attribute their origin to the more robust and reliable systems introduced by the German military in 1939. The firm AEG (now known for home appliances) first began perfecting the devices in 1935 which, when put to use, were appropriately named "Vampir," and by 1943 were mounted onto Panther tanks as telescopic rangefinders. From late 1944, when the war was all but lost, the persistent Germans had managed to mount over fifty of these sights on their tanks while also adopting "Vampir man-portable systems" on the StG44 assault rifles. Relatively speaking, production was spare and specialized with just over 300 units produced. The soldiers wielding them were called *Nachtjäger* or "night hunters." Meanwhile, already the Soviets in 1942 were beginning to test a device they called the "PAU-2," and the US military was working on night sights which they called "sniperscope" or "snooperscope."

The inventive and evocative words of yesteryear have today been squeezed into abbreviations and acronyms; the helmet-mounted scopes used by all well-equipped military units today are either called NVDs ("night vision device"), NODs ("Night optical/observation device"), or NVGs ("night-vision goggles"). These are not effective in pitch-blackness but work in light at low levels, enhancing what remains by converting near-infrared into visible contours conducive to the human eye. The resultant translated imagery comes out as a vivid emerald green, not for any chromatic compatibility to the enhancement, but because it is the least invasive of colors on the spectrum and can be viewed for extended periods. (At this point I cannot resist harking back to Nero's *smaragdus*, and the image of the Venetian noblewoman with her children with their hand-held fans with their green panes held to their faces in unison to guard against the sharp light.)

Domesticated from the military, the most widely used night vision glasses are for driving. These are typically yellow and have an anti-reflective coating that helps against headlights, streetlights, or sharp reflections off wet surfaces. The yellow tint and the protection against reflection admit better light refraction which means more available light to the naked eye.

For all the glasses in reality and fiction that bring us to a new frontier of perceptual awareness, in film they are by far more prevalent in dystopian dramas, usually as protection against inhospitable living conditions, largely extreme light, but also dust and detritus. Dystopian sci-fi is replete with ruined environments, our own or in another galaxy, of cruel and unforgiving light that makes for impassable or hard-to-penetrate conditions. It is a reminder of the balance of the burning star, the sun, the source of all life and ultimately, a longtime off, its destruction.

Or glasses may be necessary because of surgical modifications that make the eyes particularly photosensitive but acutely operative under conditions where little light is available. Such is the plight of Riddick, the anti-hero played by Vin Diesel, who first appeared in the first of the franchise, *Pitch Black* in 2000. He first comes to us in cryostasis as a prisoner on a spaceship that is forced to land on a foreign planet due to damage by microasteroids. The survivors soon find that the planet has three suns which means perpetual daylight. Riddick's glasses are more like goggles reminiscent of those used for driving in open cars in the 1920s, clamped closely to the face, permitting no intrusion of light. When his eyes are revealed, they have a blankness like the blind except that the irises, which are without pupils, have a quicksilver glow. The kicker in the story is that the survivors have arrived on the planet on the exceptional occasion of a solar eclipse of the three suns, unleashing a whole stream of nastiness from creatures normally kept in check by the presence of light. This is where Riddick, who is not only strong and ruthless but has the ability to see in darkness, comes in, and his ability to save himself and a few others along the way opens things up for a possible sequel.

In the films that followed, *The Chronicles of Riddick* (2004, not a critical success) and *Riddick* (2013, which did a little better), Riddick's eyepieces serve to confirm his position as different from the rest, physiologically and morally. They are also avatars of power held in abeyance, basic tools of containment. It is also instructive that Riddick, intended as a character in defiance of easy categories, repeatedly finds himself among those not of his kind. In *Chronicles,* for instance, the air elemental, Aereon, takes him to be a lone survivor of a thought-to-extinct race of warriors, the Furyan. In *Riddick,* we first see him as Lord Marshal of the evil Necromongers, a society of fanatics bent on destroying all humans unwilling to come into their fold. He is betrayed by them and the adventures ensue. One of the soldiers tracking him reminds his crew that "this is a man that sees in the dark," which is another way of saying that he has extraordinary powers. In the (most likely) final episode in the franchise, *Riddick: Furya*, Riddick finally comes into his own: "The power locked inside me all this time, now I know who I am. Now I'll become something they truly fear." Aristotle called the full realization of one's potential *entelekhia*, or what we now know as "entelechy," and this seems to be where Riddick is at, because now his goggles are nowhere to be seen and the silver glow of his eyes has become a shouldering blue.

It may be a little extravagant to draw too much philosophically from what is doubtlessly a piece of unapologetic commercial entertainment, it is still worth examining these pieces to consider the premises and unspoken presumptions on which they are built. The lead character's eyepieces serve as a symbol not only of his strength but his destiny and his curse, that he cannot live under all conditions, and now he is free of them and his power is unfettered. Translated into everyday language, we are waiting for when the prosthesis is no longer a clumsy addon, the thing dangled on the body, but when it can become part of us, integrated as opposed to attached to the body. If films are an indicator of collective desire, this is what we aim for: somatic enhancements that are not detachable but embedded into our physical substance.

When they began to be used in the late thirteenth century, glasses were surely viewed as futuristic, an oddity, curio. This may give us pause. Until then, for tens if not hundreds of thousands of years, humans had never worn things on their noses that improved their failing vision. Until then, there had been less reason for them, or for fewer people to avail themselves of them given the scant availability of reading matter. As one of those curious symmetries of history, all of this changed in a relatively short space of time with the introduction of movable type in the mid-fifteenth century by Johannes Gutenberg. (Although it was in the Song dynasty in China around 1040 that this kind of printing, using porcelain components, that this technique began.) The sudden flush of reading material would have exposed countless individuals to the fact that they could not see as well as they had thought, and which duly necessitated its rectification. Those weird, pretentious, ungainly contraptions sitting on the edge of the nose would rapidly be desirable, sought out, and in no great interval of time, an unremarkable item of everyday life.

One history of technology is the normalization of the remarkable over which is a new layer of the astonishing until it too becomes a matter of course. Glasses, once the specialty-crafted artifact cherished by the few that could afford them, are now available in shops where you buy chewing gum. And despite a healthy and lucrative market of prestige items, the mainstreaming of glasses also diminished their desirability.

As I have indicated many times already, glasses are not for everyone. Contact lenses have been commercially available since the 1950s and soft lenses since 1959, and they are a revelation to anyone who wants to be liberated from the encumbrances of frames and lenses. The eyes and nose can breathe free as when you were young. As anyone who has worn them knows, they are a solution with any number of limitations, including their fragility and the need to be cleaned when they fall out if you do not want to risk infection. Sudden movements are not the friends of contacts, and you definitely couldn't wear them to your next rave party without the risk of a lousy end to the evening. Be careful of being swept off your feet by an ardent lover or convulsing too hard after a lengthy case of hilarity. More recently there has been the option of laser correction to the cornea, but it is not without risks, and even when successful, a large percentage of cases eventually revert back to the same condition as before. But it is an in-built solution, prosthesis free.

There is also some talk of bionic contact lenses that bring some beloved sci-fi sequences to life by overlaying the field of vision with a display that measures and gathers data on your own life screen made of infrared lights and intricate electronic circuits. Such enhancements are enabled by Wi-Fi and can be linked to attendant personal devices, be it your laptop, phone, or watch. (It would also most likely be susceptible to external surveillance and sabotage, and here we have a new movie in the making.) These new possibilities tend to catalyze the hoary debates about technology itself and whether it improves life, whom it ultimately serves, and if it creates new needs and expectations that can only be satisfied with further advances.

True enough, glasses as an invention over seven hundred years ago were a technology, but they answered a need to revert to the kind of vision enjoyed before macular degeneration. A bionic contact lens, or bionic eye for that matter, is not a reversion to a better state of being but a transformation to a new cybernetic level which may work better as fiction or a dream than in sober reality. Humans are already reasoning animals whose success depends on ordering and analyzing our environment and imposing a rational structure on it that is of greatest benefit. Superimposing yet another matrix of analysis that is finer, more penetrating, and accurate is a seductive prospect that may be beneficial in the short term, but we might stop to reflect on the social ramifications of such measures. Already glasses themselves changed the ways in which people looked at one another, in ways both subtle and patent. But while we now hotly conjecture about the rights to the limits of state surveillance, we may also be finding ourselves having to debate the capacity of some to have immediate access to information while others do not. This may not have the dimensions of the proportions of world espionage or a James Bond villain; it can be as mundane as knowing that your partner is wearing bionic lenses while you are having sex and is able to gauge your heart rate, adrenal secretions, oxygen intake, and bodily fluids. It could be that you are trying to have an old-fashioned argument with someone who has access to all manner of information literally right before their eyes.

Where does this take us? In many ways back to the beginning, which is that glasses are so tightly wound up with knowledge. "I see" is another way of saying "I understand." (Tennyson, "In Memoriam": "For knowledge is of things we see.") Glasses were invented first for the elite who safeguarded alchemical mixtures or presided over ancient and valuable texts. To distrust the bespectacled is to go back to a primitive instinct of the fear of those who know better than yourself. Once glasses presented themselves on the social scene, it made those more prescient to be seen more easily, to the great detriment of as many if not more who did not fit the mold. At least they were visible. Bionic lenses or eyes are not, although we may discern some cybernetic glow emanating from the cornea.

How acceptable that these advantages raise more questions than answers until they are put into practice. Note that the same questions did not arise upon the inception of the garden-variety glasses. When not cultivating antipathy, glasses can also cultivate trust in either being the custodian of knowledge but also trust that this is not a person inclined to do harm. Trust is the linchpin to the next generation of glasses and ocular prosthetics, which is not limited to skepticism of a potential user; it is also of yourself. One of the more lasting of Marcel Proust's observations is: "The real voyage of discovery consists in seeing new landscapes but not in having new eyes" ("La Prisonnière"). Can you trust yourself to have serenity in your life with a continuous web of additional information before your eyes? Conventional glasses sharpen the data that is there and render it comprehensible. It seems to me that there is already too much of it out there if we choose to notice without hankering for more.

CONCLUSION

An early work and one of his few novels, Arthur Miller's *Focus* (nothing to do with the film mentioned earlier) was published in the historically loaded year of 1945, at the end of the Second World War. Set in the same period, it tells of the unassuming and contented Lawrence Newman, who is a middle manager for a large firm and enjoys a quiet life living with his mother. He witnesses some anti-Semitism in his neighborhood, such as the hostility to the local store owner by the name of Finkelstein, but is largely unruffled by it, not pursuing it in the way that others do, preferring a quiet life. But when his eyes begin to deteriorate, he is compelled by his boss to get a pair of glasses, an event that upends his life. An innocent appendage to improve his work and quality of life precipitates an unexpected fate. They become the trigger for simmering social resentment to spew forth with him as one of the unwitting scapegoats, it is a poignant twist of fate for one who has lived his life in such a meekly law-abiding, untroubled way.

The style of frames he chooses is seen as a sign of him being Jewish. Uncannily, and with a self-condemnation of which he is not yet aware, Newman is the first to see this. The scene in which he first sees himself with them on is suffused with an air of dark revelation:

> A long time he stood staring at himself, at his forehead, his chin, his nose. It took many moments of detailed inspection of his parts before he could see himself as a whole. And he felt as though rising from the floor. The beating of his heart caused his head to nod slightly in rhythm. Saliva filled a little pool in his throat and he coughed. In the mirror in his bathroom he had used for nearly seven years, he was looking at what might very properly be called the face of a Jew. A Jew, in effect, had gotten into his bathroom. The glasses did just what he had feared they would do to his face, but this was worse because this was real. It was shockingly worse than at the optometrist's three weeks ago when he tried on the frames alone.[1]

His aesthetic recognition is at once a moral one of the prejudice around a social construct that orbits around the twin satellites of glasses and Jewishness.

His immediate circle, including his neighbor, Fred, whom he thought was a friend, banished him as a Jew among gentiles, conveniently forgetting the normalcy of their relations until then. The same boss who recommended them takes measures to sequester him from view from the all-view glass office that Newman had helped to introduce.

Indignantly walking out of his job of some twenty years, Newman's once placid existence is thrown into turmoil. His bourgeois comfort is taken for avarice, and his middle-brow simplicity is now seen as a cunning ruse to assimilate. In addition to the theme of the arbitrarily invidious nature of bigotry, the broader question that Miller's story asks is that if we all tend to see the world differently according to contexts, conditions, desires, and expectations, are glasses merely a physical extension of how we choose to order the world and render the way the world sees us?

Whereas glasses have commonly featured as an adjunct to disguise in comic and serious spy narratives, Miller's story is a rare case where they are the point on which the entire narrative, with all its ethical tensions, turns. It is a brilliant literary premise, if only because it is so simple and so obvious, but it is far more than a device and the novel is far less than an allegory. Allegories are full of symbols which are proxies for universals, but while this may have some relevance here, the novel also deals with the glib semantics of appearances, meanings that have been cobbled together in an arbitrary mishmash of experience and supposition, and the prejudices that ramify from both. I would have loved to have had a conversation with Miller, who was still alive in 1978 after the Vietnamese toppled the genocidal government led by Pol Pot in Cambodia which in only three years exterminated close to two million people. Cascading numbers of carnage of this kind are usually grounded in a flimsy array of standards that are meted out with callous abandon. One criterion was wearing glasses, as these marked anyone wearing them as possibly aligned to the intelligentsia and therefore an organic threat to the regime.

Don't forget that Miller was the Jew who married Marilyn Monroe. When Marilyn married Joe DiMaggio, that was an easy fit for an actress and sex symbol to pair with a celebrated baseball player. (And for the purposes of this discussion, someone who could under no circumstances excel at wearing glasses.) But marrying a big-nosed, bespectacled, intellectual (sedentary) Jew, that was another matter. Marilyn, only thirty when she married him, apparently admitted to Miller that she had grown tired of Hollywood and that she wanted a more wholesome life. She also said that she identified with Jewish people because, like her, so many were at their throats. From an outside perspective, this was heresy. Marilyn's marriage to Miller and conversion to Judaism was not quite a betrayal, but an infection by an unworthy interloper. A chief reason for Marilyn's attraction to Miller was not only his talent and intellect but the belief that his outsider status could slough her of the artificial carapace of Marilyn so that she could become more "herself." But as noble as this wish may have been in her own mind, it was built around a contradiction from the very start. She had been actively complicit in creating a fake figure for outside consumption, from Lorna Jeane Morentson to Marilyn Monroe. If she had been created by others, it was because she too had so ably facilitated it. Miller's novel, written over ten years before he married Marilyn, would prove prophetic for the way that it shows how appearances and pathology are not separate as in outer deception and inner truth but intertwined.

Without expecting it, this becomes Newman's realization. Despite openly declaring his antipathy for Jews as if to cleanse himself of the contempt he has experienced and as an assertion of this non-Jewishness, Newman finds himself becoming other, as if by some insidious cultural osmosis. His ordinary and retiring nature assumes a timidity that suggests that he has begun to internalize the perceptions that others have foisted upon him. He meets with a series of encounters that slowly make him believe that he indeed is someone different from what he once thought he was.

On the urging of his wife—who, ironically, he had first formally met in his earlier incarnation as personnel manager in the firm he left and not hired her on the same grounds that she had not looked quite the part—he attends an Antisemitic rally held by a group calling themselves the Christian Front to which his neighbor, Fred, belongs. But he fails to play along with their histrionics. Together with how he looks, not clapping along with the crowd instantly identifies him as an interloper. As he gets mobbed, he assures that he is one of them by removing his glasses: "Quickly he pulled off his glasses and turned his face for all to see. He met a hand slapping his face—a woman's hand—and he was being pushed from behind." By this time, he had not realized that the glasses were more than mere material, they were a catalyst: "'I'm not, you damned fools, I'm not!' and he realised he had his glasses raised in one hand and was pointing to them with the other."[2]

Later Newman talks to Finkelstein and offers him a handful of flimsy justifications for his attitude to Jews and the shop owner retorts: "In other words, when you look at me you don't see me."[3] Newman is drawn into the crass web of appearances and his reactions become commensurate with the way others see him. He becomes "Jewish": "the things he had done all his life as a gentile, the most innocent habits of his person, had been turned into the tokens of an alien and evil personality, a personality that was slowly, he felt, implacably been foisted upon him."[4] In the redemptive unraveling toward the end, Newman and Finkelstein are attacked by five members of the Front and only thinly escape. Newman realizes how unreflective his antisemitism had been, and when he goes to police to prepare his statement, he is asked "How many of you people live there?" He does nothing to disabuse the policeman of the presumption behind the question, for at that moment at least he is *de facto* Jewish; his appearance and his being temporarily become one.

As I write this, it is with glasses on. They aren't prescription, just from the drug store. I have various pairs lying about the house: the study pair, the kitchen pair. When I abandoned glasses around the age of twenty, I found my vision improved without the added help, and it became next to perfect. This lasted for over twenty-five years, enough time to feel comforted in the thought that nothing much would change. Then, in the space of a few months, I noticed that I was struggling to read some smaller font. I was straining my eyes and squinting, holding the page closer, putting on an extra light. Off-the-counter glasses at +0.5 intensity initially sufficed and I was still not shouldered with the ignominy of forgetting them when reading a restaurant menu or train timetable. Now the +0.5s are in the living room and are used when I watch television there. In the kitchen I manage with +1.5s, but as I sit here, I succumb to +2.0s. There's no choice.

My glasses, my family or tribe of them, that live across my home and in my workbag are now an added dimension, not just on my face and for my eyes but physically as part of my material kit for venturing out the door: my phone, my glasses. If I want to take sunglasses as well, I may need to consider pants with non-tight accommodating pockets or else a shirt or jacket with a pocket. The reliance of old age. Yet in the inevitable disappointments of time, I have the retrospective luxury of knowing that I had them much earlier in life which means I can't reasonably just associate them with senescence. Glasses bookend my life. And where I now find that in the list of life's irritations, they rate fairly low on a world scale (if that can be taken as a rational measure), I am also able to look back down the temporal telescope to the little guy with glasses. To look back on him not with sentimentality or self-pity but with compassion. I too was made to internalize my glass-eyedness and was made well aware of how they integrated into my life and changed it from others. If I was far from singular, I was still different, and as far as I can surmise it is not the inclination of children with glasses to club together as that would be too much of an admission of their difference.

I could say that for an interval of my life I had been free of them and at least I had that, like a protracted Indian summer of sight. To that, though, would be somehow to condemn the before and the after which wouldn't be that productive. Lest it be said that glasses make me ascribe more materially and mentally to the multiple modes of being, to moving, acting, reacting, perceiving. That's how best to think of them. Not in a coldly clinical way of a prosthetic correction, but as a moderator of the world to show that our vision is tied up with countless other aspects of our bodily and psychic interactions. I recall meeting up with an old school friend a few years ago who was hearing impaired already when we were teenagers to the extent that it affected his speech and caused him to have to wear what were then big hearing aids behind his ears. He confided in me that now, with his wife and two daughters, he deems it a blessing. When they begin to squabble, he can just disconnect his hearing aids and tune out.

You might be reading with glasses now as you finish this book. When you do, take a cue from my former school buddy and take them off, relish the distorted world around you, and take in the sounds. Maybe close your eyes to listen and reflect.

Time to take them off now . . .

ACKNOWLEDGMENTS

Thanks to Dan Anlezark, Huw Griffiths, and Evan Mitchell for their tips, prompts, and advice. Thanks also to the University of Sydney for their research support.

NOTES

Chapter 1

2 Pliny the Elder, *The Natural History*, Book 37, Chapter 16, trans. John Bostock and H. T. Riley (London: Taylor and Francis, 1855), https://www.perseus.tufts.edu/hopper/text?doc=Perseus%3Atext%3A1999.02.0137%3Abook%3D37%3Achapter%3D16.

3 I am grateful to Daniel Anlezark for bringing this counterfactual to my attention.

4 Graham Pullin, "Fashion Meets Discretion," in *Design Meets Disability* (Cambridge, MA: MIT Press, 2009), 13–64.

5 Ibid.

6 Cit. Stefana Sabin, *In the Blink of an Eye: A Cultural History of Spectacles*, trans. Nick Somers (London: Reaktion, 2021), 55.

Chapter 2

1 John Le Carré, *Tinker, Tailor, Soldier, Spy* (London and New York: Penguin, 1974), 27.

2 Ibid.

3 Ibid., 45.

4 *Tinker, Tailor, Soldier, Spy*, directed by Tomas Alfredson (Studio Canal, 2011).

5 "Are Harry Potter Glasses Trendy," September 3, 2024, https://www.ancientwarrior.co.uk/blogs/articles/are-harry-potter-glasses-trendy. Accessed November 8, 2024.

6 Arthur Schopenhauer, *Counsels and Maxims*, trans. T. Bailey Saunders (London: Allen and Unwin, 1904), 96–7, emphasis in the original.

Chapter 3

1 "Neo's Cool and So are His Shades," *Chicago Tribune*, August 20, 2021, https://www.chicagotribune.com/2003/05/04/neos-cool-and-so-are-his-shades/. Accessed November 7, 2024.

2 "Why Does U2's Bono Always Wear Coloured Glasses?," *Smooth Radio*, November 10, 2021, https://www.smoothradio.com/news/music/why-does-u2s-bono-wear-glasses. Accessed December 14, 2024.

3 "Venice Put on a Show(s) – Ancient Designer Sunglasses, a Playwright, a War Hero," *Venetian Cat – The Venice Blog*, June 16, 2014, https://venetiancat.blogspot.com/2014/06/venetians-put-on-show-spectacles-fit.html. Accessed November 11, 2024.

4 See Sabin, *In the Blink of an Eye*, 9.

5 "Dark Glasses are New Fad for Wear on City Streets," *Life*, May 30, 1938, 31, https://books.google.co.th/books?id=3EoEAAAAMBAJ&pg=PA31&redir_esc=y#v=onepage&q&f=false. Accessed November 14, 2024.

6 Ibid.

7 Statista, https://www.statista.com/outlook/cmo/eyewear/sunglasses/worldwide. Accessed December 2, 2024.

8 "Tom Ford," https://www.abmopticians.com/tom-ford/. Accessed November 4, 2024.

Chapter 4

1 Michael Jung, "Superman's Glasses Are Secretly More Than Just A Disguise," *Screenrant*, July 22, 2020, https://screenrant.com/superman-glasses-secret-power-disguise/. Accessed 17 November 2024.

2 Brian Cronin, "The Surprising Origins of Clark Kent's Glasses Disguise," *CBR*, March 16, 2018, https://www.cbr.com/superman-clark-kent-harold-lloyd-glasses/. Accessed 9 November.

3 Ibid.

4 Ibid.

5 "Scientists Show that a 'Superman' Disguise could Actually Work," University of York, August 31, 2016, https://www.york.ac.uk/news-and-events/news/2016/research/superman-clark-glasses-disguise/. Accessed 11 November.

6 Ibid.

7 Lawrence Bush, "Jews in the Toy and Novelty Industry," in *Jews and American Popular Culture*, ed. Paul Buhle (London: Praeger/Bloomsbury, [2006] 2024), vol. 3, 153.

8 "History's Most Iconic Glasses," *Eyeconic*, October 23, 2017, https://blog.eyeconic.com/fashion-and-trends/historys-most-iconic-glasses.html. Accessed September 16, 2024.

Chapter 5

1 Barry Carter, "Should Sunglasses be Banned at the Poker Table?," *PokerStrategy.com*, June 14, 2022, https://www.pokerstrategy.com/news/world-of-poker/Should-sunglasses-be-banned-at-the-poker-table-_91850/. Accessed September 11, 2024.

2 Samuel Beckett, *Proust* (New York: Grove Press, 1978), 71.

3 John Puccio, "Rodrigo: Concerto de Aranjuez," *Classical Condor: Classical Music News and Reviews*, June 1, 2012, https://classicalcandor.blogspot.com/2012/06/rodrigo-concierto-de-aranjuez-hqcd.html. Accessed September 12, 2024.

4 "9 Famous Visually Impaired Women to Inspire You," https://www.orcam.com/en-us/blog/famous-visually-impaired-women-to-inspire-you?srsltid=AfmBOooK0EQBtj2l7IEmzUQsgYJsWhkJn07Lfp9ffR8SDsmjbwKMBa6A. Accessed September 11, 2024.

5 "Diane Schuur Performs with Ray Charles," https://www.youtube.com/watch?v=prTD8zWp6ck. Accessed October 19, 2024.

Chapter 6

1 "Novel Bionic Glasses Help the Blind 'See' through Sound," https://www.medicalresearch.nsw.gov.au/novel-bionic-glasses-help-the-blind-see-through-sound/. Accessed October 17, 2024.

Conclusion

1 Arthur Miller, *Focus* (London: Penguin Classics, 2009), 31–2.

2 Ibid., 177.

3 Ibid., 184.

4 Ibid., 202–3.

BIBLIOGRAPHY

Beckett, Samuel. *Proust*. New York: Grove Press, 1978.

Buhle, Paul, ed. *Jews and American Popular Culture*. London: Praeger/Bloomsbury, (2006) 2024.

Carter, Barry. "Should Sunglasses be Banned at the Poker Table?" *PokerStrategy.com*, June 14, 2022. https://www.pokerstrategy.com/news/world-of-poker/Should-sunglasses-be-banned-at-the-poker-table-_91850/.

Cronin, Brian. "The Surprising Origins of Clark Kent's Glasses Disguise." *CBR*, March 16, 2018. https://www.cbr.com/superman-clark-kent-harold-lloyd-glasses/.

Gide, André. *La Symphonie pastorale*. Paris: Nouvelle Revue Française, 1919.

Jung, Michael. "Superman's Glasses Are Secretly More Than Just A Disguise." *Screenrant*, July 22, 2020. https://screenrant.com/superman-glasses-secret-power-disguise/.

Le Carré, John. *Tinker, Tailor, Soldier, Spy*. London and New York: Penguin, 1974.

Miller Arthur. *Focus*, London: Penguin Classics, 2009.

Puccio, John. "Rodrigo: Concerto de Aranjuez." *Classical Condor: Classical Music News and Reviews*, June 1, 2012. https://classicalcandor.blogspot.com/2012/06/rodrigo-concierto-de-aranjuez-hqcd.html.

Sabin, Stefana. *In the Blink of an Eye: A Cultural History of Spectacles*. Translated by Nick Somers. London: Reaktion, 2021.

Schopenhauer, Arthur. *Counsels and Maxims*. Translated by T. Bailey Saunders. London: Allen and Unwin, 1904.

Filmography

Becoming Karl Lagerfeld, created by Isaure Pisani-Ferry, Jennifer Have, and Raphaëlle Bacqué, Disney+, 2024.
The Blues Brothers, dir. John Landis, Universal Pictures, 1980.
Bram Stoker's Dracula, dir. Francis Ford Coppola, Columbia Pictures, 1992.
Breakfast at Tiffany's, dir. Blake Edwards, Paramount Pictures, 1961.
The Breakfast Club, dir. John Hughes, Universal Pictures, 1985.
The Chronicles of Riddick, dir. David Twohy, Universal Pictures, 2004.
The Day of the Jackal, dir. Fred Zinnemann, Universal Pictures, 1973.
Dead Poets Society, dir. Peter Weir, Buena Vista Pictures, 1989.
Die Hard With a Vengeance, dir. John Tiernan, 20th Century Fox, 1995.
Ferris Bueller's Day Off, dir. John Hughes, Paramount Pictures, 1986.
Focus, dir. Glenn Ficarra and John Requa, Warner Bros., 2015.
Ghost World, dir. Terry Zwigoff, United Artists, 2001.
Good Will Hunting, dir. Gus van Sant, Miramax, 1997.
Goodbye, Mr. Chips, dir. Sam Wood, MGM, 1939.
Goodbye, Mr. Chips, dir. Herbert Ross, MGM, 1969.
The Jackal, dir. Michael Caton-Jones, Universal Pictures, 1997.
The Matrix, dir. The Wachowskis, Warner Bros., 1999.
The Matrix Resurrections, dir. Lana Wachowski, Warner Bros. Pictures, 2021.

Our Kind of Traitor, dir. Susanna White, Studio Canal, 2016.
Pitch Black, dir. David Twohy, USA Films/Universal Pictures, 2000.
The Six Million Dollar Man, produced by Kenneth Johnson, Harve Bennett Productions/Silverton Productions/Universal Television, 1973–1978.
Symphonie Pastorale, dir. Jean Delannoy, Pathé Consortium Cinéma, 1946.
Reservoir Dogs, dir. Quentin Tarantino, Miramax, 1992.
Riddick, dir. David Twohy, Universal Pictures/Entertainment One, 2013.
Riddick: Furya, dir. David Twohy, One Race Films, 2025.
Risky Business, dir. Paul Brickman, Warner Bros., 1983.
Skyfall, dir. Sam Mendes, Sony Pictures, 2012.
Spectre, dir. Sam Mendes, Sony Pictures, 2015.
Star Trek: The Next Generation, created by Gene Roddenberry, Paramount Television 1987–1994.
Superman, dir. Richard Donner, Columbia-EMI-Warner, 1978.
Tinker, Tailor, Soldier, Spy, dir. Tomas Alfredson, Studio Canal, 2011.
To Kill a Mockingbird, dir. Robert Mulligan, Universal, 1962.
The Wild One, dir. László Benedek, Columbia Pictures, 1953.

Web Sources Not Otherwise Cited

"9 Famous Visually Impaired Women to Inspire You." https://www.orcam.com/en-us/blog/famous-visually-impaired-women-to-inspire-you?srsltid=AfmBOooK0EQBtj2l7IEmzUQsgYJsWhkJn07Lfp9ffR8SDsmjbwKMBa6A.
"Are Harry Potter Glasses Trendy," September 3, 2024. https://www.ancientwarrior.co.uk/blogs/articles/are-harry-potter-glasses-trendy.

"Dark Glasses are New Fad for Wear on City Streets," *Life*, May 30, 1938, 31–3. https://books.google.co.th/books?id =3EoEAAAAMBAJ&pg=PA31&redir_esc=y#v=onepage&q&f =false.

"Diane Schuur performs with Ray Charles." https://www.youtube .com/watch?v=prTD8zWp6ck.

"History's Most Iconic Glasses." *Eyeconic*, October 23, 2017. https://blog.eyeconic.com/fashion-and-trends/historys-most -iconic-glasses.html.

"Neo's Cool and so are His Shades." *Chicago Tribune*, August 20, 2021. https://www.chicagotribune.com/2003/05/04/neos-cool -and-so-are-his-shades/.

"Novel Bionic Glasses Help the Blind 'See' through Sound." https:// www.medicalresearch.nsw.gov.au/novel-bionic-glasses-help-the -blind-see-through-sound/.

"Scientists Show that a 'Superman' Disguise could Actually Work." University of York, August 31, 2016. https://www.york.ac.uk/ news-and-events/news/2016/research/superman-clark-glasses -disguise/.

Statista. https://www.statista.com/outlook/cmo/eyewear/ sunglasses/worldwide.

"Venice Put on a Show(s) – Ancient Designer Sunglasses, a Playwright, a War Hero." *Venetian Cat – The Venice Blog*, June 16, 2014. https://venetiancat.blogspot.com/2014/06/venetians -put-on-show-spectacles-fit.html.

"Why Does U2's Bono Always Wear Coloured Glasses?." *Smooth Radio*, November 10, 2021. https://www.smoothradio.com/ news/music/why-does-u2s-bono-wear-glasses.

INDEX

Page numbers in italics refer to figures.

BLACKFACE

An Essential Non-Fiction Book of 2021, *New Statesman*
12 Best Non-Fiction Books About Black Identity and History, *Book Riot*
Book of the Week, *Times Higher Education*
2022 Prose Awards Finalist, Media and Cultural Studies Category

"A truly eye-opening, defiant, must-read."

West End Best Friend

"Wide-ranging and hard-hitting . . . a passionate, well-informed, and gripping read . . . another triumph for Object Lessons."

New York Journal of Books

"Examines Hollywood's painful, enduring ties to racist performances."

Variety

"Sharp . . . in explicitly laying out the history and costs of blackface performance, [Ayanna Thompson] fully meets her stated aim of offering an accessible book that constitutes part of an ongoing 'arc toward justice.'"

Times Higher Education

BURGER

"*Burger* draws on an accessible combination of history and pop culture to reconsider America's obsession with the molded-ground-beef sandwich . . . [It] explore[s] alternative modes of offering cultural critique, pushing against traditional divisions between academic and popular writing, and between history and critique, in search of new, more palatable forms of packaging the unsettling stories behind the Anglo-American diet."

Humanimalia

"*Burger* is a work of advocacy as well as literature and cultural analysis."

New Orleans Review

"Best known for her groundbreaking *The Sexual Politics of Meat*, Adams would seem the least likely person to write about hamburgers with her philosophically lurid antipathy to carnivory. But if the point is to deconstruct this iconic all-American meal, then she is the woman for the job."

Times Higher Education

Burger is a small book with a big punch . . . Adams approaches her topic as an animal rights advocate as well as a feminist . . . In this way, taking into account the lives of cows, as well as women, Adams convincingly explores the 'violence at the heart of the hamburger.'"

NPR: 13.7 Cosmos and Culture

It's tempting to say that *Burger* is a literary meal that fills the reader's need, but that's the essence of Adams' quick, concise, rich exploration of the role this meat (or meatless) patty has played in our lives."

PopMatters

Based on meticulous, and comprehensive, research, Adams has packed a stunning, gripping exposé into these few pages—one that may make you rethink your relationship with this food. Five stars."

San Francisco Book Review

CAT

Rebecca van Laer's *Cat* is encyclopedia entry and memoir in one, dabbling in the general history and domestication of cats, and the specific history of her cats and the lives they have lived . . . When tragedy strikes, she shares the raw edges of her sadness and anxiety with a vulnerability any animal lover will appreciate."

Shelf Awareness

For anyone who's ever watched a cat nap in sunlight and felt something stir—a reading experience both gentle and sharp."

Chronogram

Cat is a quick but deeply satisfying read. It's not just charming, or informative, or funny, or well-researched—it's also beautifully written, with lines and paragraphs that sing with their own music."

Hippocampus Magazine

DOLL

“jaw dropping.”

Is This Mutton?

“[Hart’s] observations about how dolls are emotional vectors—simultaneously objects of scorn and adoration—are revelatory and relatable.”

Brevity

“a fascinating personal and public exploration of the deeper meanings behind the plastic, polymer, and porcelain playthings that still shape American girlhood.”

Susan Shapiro, New York Times bestselling author of *Unhooked, Five Men Who Broke My Heart,* and *Barbie: Sixty Years of Inspiration*

“*Doll* is a heartfelt, intimate, and clever study of objects that terrify some and thrill others . . . giving us new perspective on these tiny, fragile mirrors.”

Allison Horrocks, co-host of the *Dolls of Our Lives* (formerly titled *American Girls Podcast*)

HIGH HEEL

Best Fifteen Books of March 2019, *Refinery29*
Best Nonfiction Books of 2019, *Paste Magazine*

> "[B]risk, readable . . . Brennan circles around the shoes from all angles, and her brief chapters add up to a kaleidoscopic view of feminine public existence, both wide-ranging and thoughtful."
>
> *Jezebel*

> "*High Heel* is poetry in prose, and while a serious work about the shoe in worldwide history and contemporary culture, it sounds more rhythmic, like poetry in motion."
>
> *San Francisco Book Review*

> "a properly modern consideration of what is at stake and it uses thoroughly intriguing methods of inquiry to approach a well-balanced lack of resolution."
>
> *PopMatters*

"From Cinderella's glass slippers to Carrie Bradshaw's Manolo Blahniks, Summer Brennan deftly analyzes one of the world's most provocative and sexualized fashion accessories in *High Heel* . . . Told in 150 vignettes that alternately entertain and educate, disturb and depress, the book ruminates on the ways in which society fetishizes, celebrates, and demonizes the high heel as well as the people, primarily women, who wear them . . . Whether you see high heels as empowering or a submission to patriarchal gender roles (or land somewhere in between), you'll likely never look at a pair the same way again after reading *High Heel*."

Longreads

"*High Heel* is thought-provoking meditation on what it means to move through the world as a woman. Brennan's book, written in very small sections, is short, but powerful enough to completely change your world view."

Refinery29

HOOD

"[I]n many ways *Hood* isn't about hoods at all. It's about what—and who—is under the hood. It's about the hooding, the hooders and the hoodees . . . [and] identity, power and politics . . . Kinney's book certainly reveals the complex history of the hood in America."

London Review of Books

“From executioners in modern-day Florida, to the Ku Klux Klan, to ‘hug a hoodie’ Cameron—this scholarly study explores a complicated cultural history . . . [Kinney’s] argument about the connection between hoods and power is a strong one . . . The book is at its best on the connections between hoods and marginalized communities.”

The Guardian

“[S]hort but ambitious . . . This provocative [book] . . . raises more questions than it seeks to answer—but that’s fitting when the issues it discusses are still so urgent and so open.”

Times Literary Supplement

“In spry and intelligent prose, Alison Kinney tours the many uses of the hood in human culture, exploring seemingly unconnected byways and guiding the reader through some surprising connections. The ubiquitous hood, she shows, is an artifact of human relationships with power, the state, and one another. By the end of my time with *Hood*, I had laughed out loud, sighed in exasperation, and felt by turns both furious and proud.”

Rebecca Onion, *Slate Magazine*

HYPHEN

"The hyphen . . . has inspired not one great book but two: *Meet Mr. Hyphen (And Put Him in His Place,* a classic by Edward N. Teall, published in 1937, and *Hyphen*, by Pardis Mahdavi, which came out in 2021."

Mary Norris, *The New Yorker*

"Mahdavi's compelling histories offer guidance for a way out of a struggle that binds us all within so many unhelpful and frankly boring binaries. The book rules."

The Stranger

SEWER

"Get ready to dive into the wondrous underworld of waste . . . It's perfect for the fatberg fan in your life."

Mental Floss

"Hester goes deep on a topic that few relish[—]the inner workings of wastewater infrastructure—all to answer questions of how human habits are reshaping the environment, and what needs to change."

Bloomberg CityLab

Takes readers on a journey underground to the meandering pipes and waterways underneath us where waste ferments and disease percolates. The oft-forgotten and hidden-but-so-necessary infrastructure below us has deep implications for urbanization, public health, infrastructure, ecology, and sustainability, not to mention our future."

Architect's Newspaper

SOUVENIR

Souvenir, a sweet new book by Rolf Potts, is a little gem (easily tucked into a jacket pocket) filled with big insights . . . *Souvenir* explores our passions for such possessions and why we are compelled to transport items from one spot to another."

Forbes

Souvenir offers ideas about what may be in play when we seek mementos . . . In the end, *Souvenir* suggests that the meaning of a keepsake is not fixed (its importance to the owner can change over time) and that its significance is bound up in the traveler's identity."

The New York Times

"Readers of this little treatise will never look at souvenirs the same way again. Five stars."

San Francisco Book Review

"A treasure trove of . . . fascinating deep dives into the history of travel keepsakes . . . [T]he book, as do souvenirs themselves, speaks to the broader issues of time, memory, adventure, and nostalgia."

The Boston Globe

STICKER

"Hoke . . . offers up an evocative reflection on queerness, race, and his hometown of Charlottesville, VA, in this conceptual 'memoir in 20 stickers.'"

Publishers Weekly

"Hoke's book uses stickers to chronicle everything from queer identity to the recent history of Charlottesville, Virginia—all of which should make this a book that sticks with you long after you've read it. (Pun intended, oh yes.)"

Volume 1 Brooklyn

“Hoke’s keenly constructed memoir-in-essays is really a memoir-in-stickers, from the glow-in-the-dark stars and coveted Lisa Frank unicorns of childhood to a Pixies decal from his teenage years.”

Electric Lit

“*Sticker* is a trove of Millennial nostalgia. Its uniqueness lies not only in Hoke’s unabashed storytelling but also in its critical analysis of American current events and its brutal honesty about a city rooted in racism . . . Hoke’s writing is blunt and honest, and *Sticker* is a collection worth keeping.”

Nicole Yurcaba, *Southern Review of Books*

STROLLER

The Best Books of 2022, *New Yorker*

“For Morgan, strollers aren’t just tools we use, or products we buy; they’re dense symbols, with no single or settled meaning, of our relationships to parenting.”

The New Yorker

VEIL

Slim but formidable."

London Review of Books

Rafia Zakaria, journalist and author, unravels the complex nexus of attitudes, policies, and histories revolving around this object in her fascinating new book, *Veil*. She demonstrates how the object can serve as a moral delineator, a disciplinary measure, a signifier of goodness, or as a means to subvert or rebel social norms. Through personal narratives and detailed analysis of various social and political conditions Zakaria offers an engaging and nuanced assessment of the veil in the contemporary context."

New Books Network

I admired Rafia Zakaria's *Veil* months even before I read it . . . Her engaging prose is just what I hoped to find inside this little book, which is composed of short vignettes on the veil rather than a sustained philosophical treaty."

Reading Religion